Pocket
Companion for
Physical
Examination
and
Health
Assessment

Pocket Companion for
Physical Examination and Health Assessment

■ Carolyn Jarvis, RN, C, MSN, FNP

Adjunct Assistant Professor of Nursing
School of Nursing
Illinois Wesleyan University
Bloomington, Illinois
and
Family Nurse Practitioner
Chestnut Health Systems
Bloomington, Illinois

W.B. SAUNDERS COMPANY
A Division of Harcourt Brace & Company
Philadelphia London Toronto
Montreal Sydney Tokyo

W.B. SAUNDERS COMPANY
A Division of
Harcourt Brace & Company

The Curtis Center
Independence Square West
Philadelphia, Pennsylvania 19106

Library of Congress Cataloging-in-Publication Data

Jarvis, Carolyn.
    Pocket companion for physical examination and health assessment /
Carolyn Jarvis. — 1st ed.
    p.   cm.
    ISBN 0-7216-4669-7
    1. Physical diagnosis — Handbooks, manuals, etc.   2. Medical
history taking — Handbooks, manuals, etc.   I. Title.
RC76.J374   1993
616.07'54 — dc20   92-23447

Pocket Companion for
PHYSICAL EXAMINATION AND
HEALTH ASSESSMENT   ISBN   0-7216-4669-7

Printed in the United States of America.

Last digit is the print number: 9   8   7   6   5   4   3   2

About the Author

Carolyn Jarvis received her B.S.N. cum laude from the University of Iowa in 1968 and her M.S.N. from Loyola University (Chicago) in 1974. She has taught physical assessment and critical care nursing at Rush University (Chicago), University of Missouri (Columbia), and University of Illinois (Urbana), and she currently serves as Adjunct Assistant Professor at Illinois Wesleyan University in Bloomington.

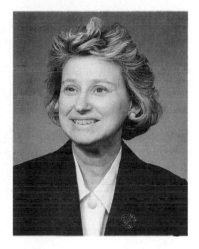

Ms. Jarvis is a recipient of the University of Missouri's Superior Teaching Award and has taught physical assessment to hundreds of baccalaureate students and nursing professionals, has held 150 countinuing education seminars, and is the author of numerous articles and textbook contributions.

Ms. Jarvis has maintained a clinical practice for over 20 years in advanced practice roles—first as a cardiovascular clinical specialist in various critical care settings and, for the last 12 years, as a certified family nurse practitioner in primary care. She is currently a nurse practitioner at Chestnut Health Systems, Bloomington, Illinois.

Preface

The *Pocket Companion for Physical Examination and Health Assessment* is designed for two uses — for those who need a practical clinical reference and for those acquiring beginning assessment skills.

First, the PC is intended as an adjunct to Jarvis's *Physical Examination and Health Assessment*. The PC is a memory prompt for those who have studied physical assessment and wish a reminder when in the clinical area. The PC has all the essentials: health history points, exam steps for each body system, normal vs. abnormal findings, heart sounds, lung sounds, neuro checks. The PC is useful when you forget a step in the exam sequence, when you wish to be sure your assessment is complete, when you need to review those findings that are normal versus abnormal, or when you are faced with an unfamiliar technique or a new clinical area. Its portable size and binding make it perfect for a lab coat pocket or community health bag.

Second, the *Pocket Companion* is an independent primer of basic assessment skills. It is well suited to programs offering a beginning assessment course covering well people of all ages. The PC has the complete steps to perform a health history and physical examination on a well person. It includes pertinent developmental content for pediatric, pregnant, and aging adult groups. Although the description of each exam step is stated very concisely, there is enough information given to study and learn exam techniques. However, since there is no room in the PC for theories, principles or detailed explanations, students using the PC as a beginning text must have a thorough didactic presentation of assessment methods as well as tutored practice.

For those times when readers need detailed coverage of a particular technique or finding, it is easily found through numerous cross references to pages in *Physical Examination and Health Assessment.*

As you thumb through the PC, note these features:

- Health history and exam steps are concise yet complete
- Method of examination is clear, orderly, and easy to follow
- Abnormal findings are described briefly in a column adjacent to the normal range of findings
- Tables are presented at the ends of chapters to fully illustrate important information
- Selected Transcultural Considerations highlight this important aspect of a health assessment
- Nursing Diagnoses are provided fully for each region or system being assessed
- Developmental content includes age specific information for pediatric, pregnant, and aging adult groups

- Summary checklists for each chapter form a cue card of exam steps to remember
- Integration of the complete physical examination is presented in Chapter 20

- Sample Recording in Chapter 20 illustrates the documentation of normal findings
- Selected artwork from *Physical Examination and Health Assessment* illustrates the pertinent anatomy.

Acknowledgments

Thanks to Michael J. Brown, Editor-in-Chief, for his encouragement and unfailing support in guiding this project from start to finish. Thanks to Suzanne Schiding in Production Services at Progressive Typographers for her careful, exacting management of both text and art. Thanks, too, to Joan Sinclair, Production Manager at W. B. Saunders, for attentive monitoring of all aspects of the *Pocket Companion*.

I am grateful to Pat Thomas, whose stunning art from *Physical Examination and Health Assessment* is reproduced so beautifully in the *Pocket Companion* and who contributed new art just for this book. I am grateful also to Margaret Andrews, PhD, RN, whose contributions to the Transcultural Considerations sections in *Physical Examination and Health Assessment* have been selected and reproduced here in the *Pocket Companion*.

Carolyn Jarvis

Table of Contents

1 The Interview and the Health History

The health history is important in beginning to identify the person's health strengths and problems and as a bridge to the next step in data collection, the physical examination.

The health history collects *subjective data*, what the person says about himself or herself. This is the first and the best chance a person has to tell you what *he* or *she* perceives the health state to be.

External Factors

Ensure Privacy. Aim for geographic privacy—a private room. If geographic privacy is not available, "psychologic privacy" by curtained partitions may suffice as long as the person feels sure no one can overhear the conversation or interrupt.

Refuse Interruptions. You need to concentrate and to establish rapport.

Physical Environment

• Set the room temperature at a comfortable level.
• Provide sufficient lighting.
• Reduce noise
• Remove distracting objects.
• Place the distance between you at 4 to 5 feet (twice an arm's length).
• Arrange equal-status seating. Both you and the client should be comfortably seated at eye level. Avoid sitting behind a desk or bedside table placed so that it looks like a barrier.
• Avoid standing.

There are three phases to each interview: an introduction, a working phase, and a termination.

Introducing the Interview

Address the person, using his or her surname. Introduce yourself and state your role in the agency (if you are a student, say so). If you are gathering a complete history, give the reason for this interview.

The Working Phase

The working phase is the data gathering phase. It involves your questions to the client and your response to what the client has said. There are two types of questions: open-ended and closed or direct. Each type has a different place and function in the interview.

Open-Ended Questions

The open-ended question asks for narrative information. It states the topic to be discussed but only in general terms. Use it to begin the interview, to introduce a new section of questions, and whenever the person introduces a new topic. An example would be, "Tell me why you have come here today."

Closed or Direct Questions

Closed or direct questions ask for specific information. They elicit a short, one- or two-word answer, a yes or no, or a forced choice. Use direct questions after the person's narrative to fill in any details he or she may have omitted. Also use direct questions when you need many specific facts, such as when asking about past health problems or during the review of systems.

Responses

As the person talks, your role is to encourage free expression, but to not let the person wander.

Facilitation. These responses encourage the client to say more, to continue with the story, e.g., "mm-hmm," "go on," "continue," "uh-huh," or simply nodding "yes."

Silence. Silence communicates that the person has time to think, to organize what he or she wishes to say without interruption from you. Silence also gives you a chance to observe the person unobtrusively and to note nonverbal cues.

Reflection. This response echoes the client's words. It repeats part of what the person has just said. It focuses further attention on a specific phrase and helps the person continue in his or her own way.

Empathy. An empathic response recognizes a feeling and puts it into words. It names the feeling and allows the expression of it. When the empathic response is used, the client feels accepted and can deal with the feeling openly. Empathic responses are, "This must be very hard for you," or just placing your hand on the person's arm.

Clarification. Use the clarification response when the person's word choice is ambiguous or confusing,

e.g., "Tell me what you mean by 'bad blood.'"

Confrontation. In this case, you have observed a certain action, feeling, or statement, and you now focus the person's attention on it. This may focus on a discrepancy: "You say it doesn't hurt, but when I touch you here, you grimace." Or, it may focus on the person's affect: "You look sad," or "You sound angry."

Interpretation. This response is not based on direct observation (as is confrontation) but on your inference or conclusion. Interpretation links events, makes associations, or implies cause: "It seems that every time you feel the stomach pain, you have had some kind of stress in your life."

Explanation. With these statements, you share factual and objective information. This may be for orientation to the agency setting: "Your dinner comes at 5:30 P.M." or it may be to explain cause: "The reason you cannot eat or drink before your blood test is that the food will change the test results."

Summary. This is a final review of what you understand the person has said. It condenses the facts and presents a survey of how you perceive the health problem or need.

Closing the Interview

The meeting should end gracefully. To ease into the closing, ask the person, e.g., "Is there anything else you would like to mention?" Give the person a final opportunity for self expression. Then give your summary or a recapitulation of what you have learned during the interview. This is a final statement of what you and the client agree the health state to be.

Ten Traps of Interviewing

Nonproductive, defeating verbal messages are messages that restrict the client's response. They are obstacles to obtaining complete data and to establishing rapport.

Providing Assurance or Reassurance. Such statements as "Now don't worry, I'm sure you will be all right" are courage builders that relieve *your* anxiety and give you a false sense of having provided comfort. For the client, however, these statements close off communication. They trivialize anxiety and effectively deny further discussion.

Giving Advice. A person describes a problem to you, ending with "What would you do?" If you answer, "If I were you, I'd . . . ," you have shifted the accountability for decision-making from the person to you. The person has not worked out his or her own solution and has learned nothing about himself or herself.

Using Authority. "Your doctor/ nurse knows best" is a response that promotes dependency and inferiority.

Using Avoidance Language. People use euphemisms, such as "passed on," to avoid reality or to hide their feelings.

Engaging in Distancing. This is the use of impersonal speech to put space between a threat and the self.

Using Professional Jargon. Use of jargon sounds exclusionary and paternalistic. You need to adjust your vocabulary to the person but should avoid sounding condescending.

Using Leading or Biased Questions. Asking such questions as "You don't smoke, do you?" implies that one answer is "better" than another.

Talking Too Much. Some examiners associate helpfulness with how much they talk. They think they have met the client's needs. Just the opposite is true.

Interrupting. Often, when you think you know what the person will say, you interrupt and cut the person off.

Using "Why" Questions. The adult's use of why questions usually implies blame and condemnation, and puts the person on the defensive.

Nonverbal Skills

Nonverbal messages that are productive and enhancing to the relationship are those that show attentiveness and unconditional acceptance. Defeating, nonproductive, nonverbal behaviors are those of inattentiveness, authority, and superiority (Table 1–1).

Table 1–1 ▶ Nonverbal Behaviors of the Interviewer	
POSITIVE	**NEGATIVE**
Appropriate professional appearance	Appearance objectionable to client
Equal status seating	Standing
Close proximity to client	Sitting behind desk, far away, turned away
Relaxed open posture	Tense posture
Leaning slightly toward person	Slouched back
Occasional facilitation gestures	Critical or distracting gestures: pointing finger, clenched fist, finger-tapping, foot-swinging, looking at watch
Facial animation, interest	Bland expression, yawning, tight mouth
Appropriate smiling	Frowning, lip biting
Maintain appropriate eye contact	Shifty, avoiding eye contact, focusing on notes
Moderate tone of voice	Strident, high-pitched tone
Moderate rate of speech	Rate too slow or too fast
Appropriate touch	Too frequent or inappropriate touch

THE HEALTH HISTORY—
THE ADULT

Biographical Data

Name, address, phone number, age, birthdate, birthplace, sex, marital status, race, ethnic origin, and occupation, usual and present.

Source of History

Reason for Seeking Care

This is a brief spontaneous statement in the person's own words that describes the reason for the visit.

Present Health or History of Present Illness

This is a chronologic record of the reason for seeking care, from the time of the onset of the symptoms until now. Start in the past when the person first noticed the symptoms and work forward to the present. Your final summary of any symptom the person has should include these *eight critical characteristics:*

1 ▶ Location. Be specific, ask the person to point to it.
2 ▶ Character or quality.
3 ▶ Quantity or severity.
4 ▶ Timing (onset, duration, frequency).
5 ▶ Setting.
6 ▶ Aggravating or relieving factors.
7 ▶ Associated factors.
8 ▶ Client's perception of what the symptom means.

Past Health

Childhood Illnesses. Measles, mumps, rubella, chicken pox, pertussis, strep throat, rheumatic fever, scarlet fever, and poliomyelitis.

Accidents or Injuries.

Serious or Chronic Illnesses. Diabetes, hypertension, heart disease, sickle cell anemia, cancer, and seizure disorder.

Hospitalizations.

Operations.

Obstetric History. The number of pregnancies (gravidity), number of deliveries in which the fetus reached viability (parity), and number of abortions.

Immunizations. All childhood immunizations (measles/mumps/rubella, polio, diphtheria/pertussis/tetanus) and were they kept up to date. Also note the last tetanus immunization, last tuberculosis skin test, and last flu shot.

Last Examination Date. The most recent physical, dental, vision, hearing, ECG, and chest x-ray examinations.

Allergies. Medication, food, environmental agent. Note reaction.

Current Medications. All prescription and over-the-counter medications including laxatives, vitamins, birth control pills, aspirin, and antacids.

Family History

The age and health or the age and cause of death of blood relatives, such as parents, grandparents, and siblings. The age and health of spouse and children. Specifically, any family history of: heart disease, high blood pressure, stroke, diabetes, blood disorders, cancer, sickle cell anemia, arthritis, allergies, obesity, alcoholism, mental illness, seizure disorder, kidney disease, or tuberculosis. Construct a family tree, or genogram, to show this information clearly and concisely (Fig. 1–1).

Review of Systems

General Overall Health State. Present weight (gain or loss, period of time, by diet or other factors), fatigue, weakness or malaise, fever, chills, and sweats or night sweats.

Skin. History of skin disease (eczema, psoriasis, hives), pigment or

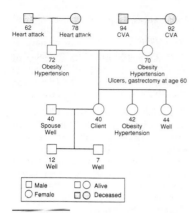

▶ Figure 1-1   A family tree, or genogram

color change, change in mole, excessive dryness or moisture, pruritus, excessive bruising, and rash or lesion. **Hair.** Recent loss, change in texture. **Nails.** Change in shape, color, or brittleness.

Health Promotion. Amount of sun exposure.

Head. Unusually frequent or severe headache, any head injury, dizziness (syncope), or vertigo.

Eyes. Difficulty with vision (decreased acuity, blurring, blind spots), eye pain, diplopia (double vision), redness or swelling, watering or discharge, and glaucoma or cataracts.

Health Promotion. Wear glasses or contacts, last vision check or glaucoma test, and ways of coping with vision loss.

Ears. Earaches, infections, discharge and its characteristics, tinnitus, or vertigo.

Health Promotion. Hearing loss, hearing aid use, effect of hearing loss on daily life, exposure to environmental noise, and method of cleaning ears.

Nose and Sinuses. Discharge and its characteristics, unusually frequent or severe colds, any sinus pain, nasal obstruction, nosebleeds, aller-

gies or hay fever, or change in sense of smell.

Mouth and Throat. Mouth pain, frequent sore throat, bleeding gums, toothache, lesion in mouth or tongue, dysphagia, hoarseness or voice change, altered taste. History of tonsillectomy.

Health Promotion. Pattern of daily dental care, use of prosthesis (dentures, bridge), and last dental checkup.

Neck. Pain, limitation of motion, lumps or swelling, enlarged or tender nodes, or goiter.

Breast. Pain, lump, nipple discharge, rash, or breast disease.

Health Promotion. Breast self-exam method and frequency.

Axilla. Tenderness, lump or swelling, or rash.

Respiratory System. History of lung diseases (asthma, emphysema, bronchitis, pneumonia, tuberculosis), chest pain with breathing, wheezing or noisy breathing, shortness of breath, how much activity produces shortness of breath, cough, sputum (color, amount), hemoptysis, and toxin or pollution exposure.

Cardiovascular. Precordial or retrosternal pain, palpitation, cyanosis, dyspnea on exertion (specify amount of exertion), orthopnea, paroxysmal nocturnal dyspnea, nocturia, edema, history of heart murmur, hypertension, coronary artery disease, or anemia.

Peripheral Vascular. Coldness, numbness and tingling, swelling of legs (time of day, activity), discoloration in hands or feet, varicose veins or complications, intermittent claudication, thrombophlebitis, or ulcers.

Health Promotion. Amount of long-term sitting or standing, habit of crossing legs at the knees, use of support hose.

Gastrointestinal. Appetite, food intolerance, dysphagia, heartburn, indigestion, pain (associated with eating), other abdominal pain, pyrosis (esophageal and stomach burning sensation with sour eructation), nausea and vomiting (character), vomiting blood, history of abdominal disease (ulcer, liver or gallbladder, jaundice, appendicitis, colitis), flatulence, frequency of bowel movements (any recent change), stool characteristics, constipation or diarrhea, black stools, rectal bleeding, or rectal conditions (hemorrhoids, fistula).

Urinary System. Frequency, urgency, nocturia (recent change), dysuria, polyuria or oliguria, hesitancy or straining, narrowed stream, urine color (cloudy or presence of blood), incontinence, history of urinary disease (kidney disease, kidney stones, urinary tract infections, prostate disease), or pain in flank, groin, suprapubic region, or low back.

Health Promotion. Use of Kegel exercises after childbirth, measures to avoid or treat urinary tract infections.

Male Genital System. Penile or testicular pain, sores or lesions, penile discharge, lumps, or hernia.

Health Promotion. Testicular self-examination.

Female Genital System. Menstrual history (age at menarche, last menstrual period, cycle and duration, amenorrhea or menorrhagia, premenstrual pain or dysmenorrhea, intermenstrual spotting), vaginal itching, discharge and its characteristics, age at menopause, menopausal signs or symptoms, or postmenopausal bleeding.

Health Promotion. Last gynecologic checkup and last Papanicolaou smear.

Sexual Health. Current sexual activity. Are the aspects of sex satisfactory to the client and partner? Any dyspareunia (for female), any changes in erection or ejaculation (for male)? Use of contraceptive? Contraceptive method satisfactory? Aware of contact with a partner who has any sexually transmitted disease (gonorrhea, herpes, Chlamydia, venereal warts, AIDS, or syphilis)?

Musculoskeletal System. History of arthritis or gout. Joint pain, stiffness, swelling (location, migratory nature), deformity, limitation of motion, or noise with joint motion. Muscle pain, cramps, weakness, gait problems, or problems with coordinated activities. Other pain (location and radiation to extremities), stiffness, limitation of motion, or history of back pain or disc disease.

Health Promotion. How much walking per day? What is the effect of limited range of motion on daily activities, such as grooming, feeding, toileting, or dressing. Are any mobility aids used?

Neurologic System. History of seizure disorder, stroke, fainting, or blackouts. Motor function: any weakness, tic or tremor, paralysis or coordination problems. Sensory function: any numbness and tingling (paresthesia). Cognitive function: any memory disorder (recent or distant, disorientation). Mental status: nervousness, mood change, depression, or history of mental health dysfunction or hallucinations.

Hematologic System. Bleeding of skin or mucous membranes, excessive bruising, lymph node swelling, exposure to toxic agents or radiation, or blood transfusion and reactions.

Endocrine System. History of diabetes or diabetic symptoms (polyuria, polydipsia, polyphagia), history of thyroid disease, intolerance to heat and cold, change in skin pigmentation or texture, excessive sweating, relationship between appetite and weight, abnormal hair distribution, nervousness, tremors, or need for hormone therapy.

Functional Assessment (Activities of Daily Living)

Functional assessment measures a person's self-care ability in the areas of physical health, activities of daily living, nutritional status, and psychosocial status. These questions provide data on the lifestyle and type of living environment to which the person is accustomed.

Self-Esteem, Self-Concept. Education (last grade completed, other significant training), financial status (income adequate for lifestyle and/or health concerns), value-belief system (religious practices and perception of personal strengths).

Activity-Exercise. A daily profile reflecting usual daily activities. Ability to perform activities of daily living (ADL). Independent or needs assistance. Able to tolerate activity, or use prostheses or mobility aids. Leisure activities enjoyed and exercise pattern (type, amount per day or week, warm-up session, body's response to exercise).

Sleep/Rest. Sleep patterns, any sleep aids.

Nutrition. Recall all food and beverages taken over the last 24 hours. Is that menu typical? Eating habits and current appetite. (Who buys food and prepares food? Are finances adequate for food? Who is present at mealtimes?) Any food allergy or intolerance. Habits: daily intake of caffeine (coffee, tea, cola drinks), alcohol ("When was your last drink of alcohol?" "How much did you drink that time?" "Have you ever had a drinking problem?"), smoking ("Do you smoke?" "At what age did you start?" "How many packs do you smoke per day?" "How many years have you smoked?"), and street drugs ("Have you ever tried any drugs such as marijuana, cocaine, amphetamines, or barbiturates?" "How often do you use these drugs?" and "How has usage affected your work or social relationships?").

Interpersonal Relationships. Social roles ("Role in your family?" "How would you say you get along with family, friends, and co-workers?") and support systems composed of family and significant others ("To whom could you go for support with a problem at work, with your health, or a personal problem?").

Coping and Stress Management. Housing and neighborhood (live alone, know neighbors, safety of area, adequate heat and utilities, access to transportation, involved in community services) and environmental health (hazards in workplace, hazards at home, use of seatbelts, geographic or occupational exposures, travel or residence in other countries). What kinds of stresses are present in life now and in the last year? Has there been any change in lifestyle or any current stress? Any steps tried to relieve stress? Has this helped?

Perception of Health

"How do you define health?" "How do you view your situation now?" "What are your concerns?" "What do you think will happen in the future?" "What are your health goals?" "What do you expect from us as nurses, physicians, (other health care providers)?"

For more information on the health history of infants and children, older adults, and cultural assessment, see Jarvis: *Physical Examination and Health Assessment,* **pp. 83–99.**

CHAPTER

2 Mental Status

Mental status is a person's emotional and cognitive functioning. Optimal functioning aims toward simultaneous life satisfaction in work, in caring relationships, and within the self.

Mental status cannot be scrutinized directly like the characteristics of skin or heart sounds. Its functioning is *inferred* through assessment of an individual's behaviors:

Consciousness: being aware of one's own existence, feelings, and thoughts, and aware of the environment.

Language: using the voice to communicate one's thoughts and feelings.

Mood and affect: both of these elements deal with prevailing feelings. Mood is a prolonged display of feelings that colors the whole emotional life; affect is a temporary expression of feelings.

Orientation: awareness of the objective world in relation to the self.

Attention: the power of concentration, the ability to focus on one specific thing without being distracted.

Memory: the ability to note and store experiences and perceptions for later recall. *Recent* memory evokes day-to-day events; *remote* memory brings up many years' worth of experiences.

Abstract reasoning: pondering a deeper meaning beyond the concrete and literal.

Thought process: the *way* a person thinks, the logical train of thought.

Thought content: *what* the person thinks; specific ideas, beliefs, the use of words.

Perceptions: an awareness of objects through any of the five senses.

THE MENTAL STATUS EXAMINATION

The full mental status examination is a systematic check of emotional and cognitive functioning. The steps described here, though, rarely need to be taken in their entirety. Usually, you can assess mental status through the context of the health history interview. During that time, keep in mind the four main headings of mental status assessment:

Appearance,

Behavior,

Cognition, and

Thought processes,

or A, B, C, T.

In every mental status examination, note these factors from the health history that could affect your findings:

- any known illnesses or health problems, such as alcoholism, or chronic renal disease;
- current medications whose side effects may cause confusion or depression;
- the usual educational and behavioral level—note that factor as the normal baseline, and do not expect performance on the mental status examination to exceed it;
- responses to personal history questions, indicating current stress, social interaction patterns, and sleep habits.

Appearance

Posture is erect and **position** is relaxed.

Body movements are voluntary, deliberate, coordinated, and smooth and even.

Dress is appropriate for setting, season, age, gender, and social group. Clothing fits and is put on appropriately.

Grooming and hygiene reveal the person to be clean and well-groomed, hair neat and clean, women with moderate or no make-up, men clean shaven, or beard or moustache is well-groomed. Nails are clean (though some jobs leave nails chronically dirty). Note: A disheveled appearance in a previously well-groomed person is significant. Use care in interpreting clothing that is disheveled, bizarre, or in poor repair because this sometimes may reflect the person's economic status or a deliberate fashion trend.

Behavior

Level of Consciousness. The person is alert, aware of stimuli from the environment and within the self, and responds appropriately. (Table 2–1).

Facial Expression. The look is appropriate to the situation and changes appropriately with the topic. There is comfortable eye contact unless precluded by cultural norm (e.g., Native American).

Speech. *Quality*—The person makes laryngeal sounds effortlessly and shares conversation appropriately.

The *pace* of the conversion is moderate, and stream of talking is fluent.

Articulation (ability to form words) is clear and understandable.

Word choice is effortless and appropriate to educational level. The person completes sentences, occasionally pausing to think.

Mood Affect. Determine this by body language and facial expression, and by asking directly, "How do you feel today," or "How do you usually feel?" The mood should be appropriate to the person's place and condition and change appropriately with topics. The person is willing to cooperate with you.

Cognitive Functions

Orientation. You can discern orientation through the course of the interview. Assess:

- *Time: day of week, date, year, season.*
- *Place: where person lives, present location, type of building, name of city and state.*
- *Person: own name, age, who examiner is, type of worker.*

Many hospitalized people normally have trouble with the exact date but are fully oriented to other items.

Attention Span. Check the person's ability to concentrate by noting whether he or she completes a thought without wandering. Note any distractibility or difficulty attending to you, or give a series of directions to follow and note the correct sequence of behaviors. Note that attention span commonly is impaired in people who are anxious, fatigued, or drug intoxicated.

Recent Memory. Assess recent memory in the context of the interview by the 24-hour diet recall.

Remote Memory. In the context of the interview, ask the person

Table 2-1 ► Levels of Consciousness

These terms are commonly used in clinical practice. They spread over a continuum from full alertness to deep coma. The terms are qualitative and therefore are not always reliable. (A *quantitative* tool that serves the same purpose and eliminates ambiguity is the Glasgow Coma Scale in Chapter 16.) These terms are widely accepted, however, and are useful as long as all co-workers agree on definitions and are consistent in their application.

To increase clarity when using these terms, also record:

1. the level of stimulus used, ranging progressively from
   a. name called in normal tone of voice.
   b. name called in loud voice
   c. light touch on person's arm.
   d. vigorous shake of shoulder.
   e. pain applied.

2. the person's response
   a. amount and quality of movement.
   b. presence and coherence of speech.
   c. opens eyes and makes eye contact.

3. what the person does on cessation of your stimulus.

ALERT

Awake or readily aroused, oriented, fully aware of external and internal stimuli, and responds appropriately, conducts meaningful interpersonal interactions.

LETHARGIC

Somnolent, drifts off to sleep when not stimulated, can be aroused to name when called in normal voice but looks drowsy, responds appropriately to questions or commands but thinking seems slow and fuzzy, inattentive, loses train of thought, spontaneous movements are decreased.

OBTUNDED

(Transitional state between lethargy and stupor; some sources omit this level.)

Sleeps most of time, difficult to arouse—needs loud shout or vigorous shake, acts confused when aroused, converses in monosyllables, speech may be mumbled and incoherent, requires constant stimulation for even marginal cooperation.

STUPOR OR SEMI-COMA

Spontaneously unconscious, responds only to vigorous shake or pain, has appropriate motor response (i.e., withdraws hand to avoid pain), otherwise can only groan, mumble, or move restlessly, reflex activity persists.

COMA

Completely unconscious, no response to pain nor to any external or internal stimuli (e.g., when suctioned, will not try to push the catheter away), light coma has some reflex activity but not purposeful movement, deep coma has no motor response.

ACUTE CONFUSIONAL STATE (DELIRIUM)

Clouding of consciousness (dulled cognition, impaired alertness), inattentive, incoherent conversation, impaired recent memory and confabulatory for recent events, often agitated and has visual hallucinations, disoriented, with confusion worse at night when environmental stimuli are decreased.

(Adapted from Strub RL, and Black FW: The Mental Status Examination in Neurology, 2nd. ed. Philadelphia, FA Davis, 1985, with permission.)

verifiable past events, e.g., describe past health, first job, birthday and anniversary dates, and historical events.

Judgment. To assess judgment in the context of the interview, note what the person says about job plans, social or family obligations, and plans for the future. Also ask the person to describe the rationale for personal health care, and how he or she decided about complying with prescribed health regimens. The person's actions and decisions should be realistic.

Thought Processes and Perceptions

Thought Processes. Ask yourself, "Does this person make sense? Can I follow what the person is saying?" The *way* a person thinks should be logical, goal directed, coherent, and relevant. The person should complete a thought.

Thought Content. *What* the person says should be consistent and logical.

Perceptions. The person should be consistently aware of reality. The perceptions should be congruent with yours. Ask the following questions:

- How do people treat you?
- Do other people talk about you?
- Do you feel as if you are being watched, followed, or controlled?
- Is your imagination very active?
- Have you heard your name when alone?

Screen for Suicidal Thoughts. When the person expresses feelings of sadness, hopelessness, despair or grief, it is important to assess any possible risk of physical harm to himself or herself. Begin with more general questions. If you hear affirmative answers, continue with more specific questions:

- Have you ever felt so blue you thought of hurting yourself?

- Do you feel like hurting yourself now?
- Do you have a plan to hurt yourself?
- What would happen if you were dead?
- How would other people react if you were dead?

Do not skip these questions if you have the slightest clue that they are appropriate. You may be the only health professional to pick up clues to suicide risk. You are responsible for encouraging the person to talk about suicidal thoughts. Sometimes you cannot prevent a suicide when someone really wishes to kill himself or herself. The majority of people are ambivalent, however, and you can buy time, so that the person can be helped to find an alternate solution to the situation.

Supplemental Mental Status Examination

The Mini-Mental State Examination is a simplified scored form of the cognitive functions of the mental status examination (Folstein, et al, 1975). It is quick and easy, includes a standard set of only 11 questions, and requires only 5 to 10 minutes to administer. It is useful for both initial and serial measurement, so you can demonstrate worsening or improvement of cognition over time and with treatment. The Mini-Mental State Examination concentrates only on cognitive functioning, not on mood or thought processes. It is a valid detector of organic disease, and thus, is a good screening tool for detecting dementia and delirium.

The maximum score on the test is 30; an average score of 27 is normal. Scores below 20 occur with dementia and delirium. (Table 2–2)

For more information on abnormalities of mood and affect, organic brain syndromes, substance use disorders, schizophrenia, mood disorders, anxiety disorders, see Jarvis: *Physical Examination and Health Assessment,* **pp. 114–124.**

Table 2-2 ▶ Mini-Mental State Examination

Patient _____   Examiner _____   Date _____

Maximum Score	Score	
		ORIENTATION
5	( )	What is the (year) (season) (day) (month)?
5	( )	Where are we: (state) (country) (town) (hospital) (floor)?
		REGISTRATION
3	( )	Name 3 objects: 1 second to say each. Then ask the patient all 3 after you have said them. Give 1 point for each correct answer. Then repeat them until he learns all 3. Count trials and record. Trials _____
		ATTENTION AND CALCULATION
5	( )	Serial 7's. 1 point for each correct. Stop after 5 answers. Alternatively spell "world" backwards.
		RECALL
3	( )	Ask for 3 objects repeated above. Give 1 point for each correct.
		LANGUAGE
9	( )	Name a pencil, and watch (2 points). Repeat the following "No ifs, ands, or buts." (1 point)
		Follow a 3-stage command:
		"Take a paper in your right hand, fold it in half, and put it on the floor." (3 points)
		Read and obey the following:
		CLOSE YOUR EYES (1 point)
		Write a sentence (1 point)
		Copy design (1 point)
_____		Total Score
		ASSESS level of consciousness along a continuum

Alert   Drowsy   Stupor   Coma

Instructions for Administration of Mini-Mental State Examination

ORIENTATION

(1) Ask for the date. Then ask specifically for parts omitted, e.g., "Can you also tell me what season it is?" One point for each correct.

(2) Ask in turn, "Can you tell me the name of this hospital?" (town, country, etc.). One point for each correct.

REGISTRATION

Ask the patient if you may test his memory. Then say the names of 3 unrelated objects, clearly and slowly, about one second for each. After you have said all 3, ask him to repeat them. This first repetition determines his score (0–3) but keep saying them until he can repeat all 3, up to 6 trials. If he does not eventually learn all 3, recall cannot be meaningfully tested.

ATTENTION AND CALCULATION

Ask the patient to begin with 100 and count backwards by 7. Stop after 5 subtractions (93, 86, 79, 72, 65). Score the total number of correct answers.

If the patient cannot or will not perform this task, ask him to spell the word "world" backward. The score is the number of letters in correct order, e.g. dlrow = 5, dlorw = 3.

Table 2-2 ▶ Mini-Mental State Examination *Continued*

RECALL

Ask the patient if he can recall the 3 words you previously asked him to remember. Score 0-3.

LANGUAGE

Naming: Show the patient a wrist watch and ask him what it is. Repeat for pencil. Score 0-2.

Repetition: Ask the patient to repeat the sentence after you. Allow only one trial. Score 0 or 1.

3-Stage Command: Give the patient a piece of plain blank paper and repeat the command. Score 1 point for each part correctly executed.

Reading: On a blank piece of paper print the sentence "Close your eyes" in letters large enough for the patient to see clearly. Ask him to read it and do what it says. Score 1 point only if he actually closes his eyes.

Writing: Give the patient a blank piece of paper and ask him to write a sentence for you. Do not dictate a sentence, it is to be written spontaneously. It must contain a subject and verb and be sensible. Correct grammar and punctuation are not necessary.

Copying: On a clean piece of paper, draw intersecting pentagons, each side about 1 in., and ask him to copy it exactly as it is. All 10 angles must be present and 2 must intersect to score 1 point. Tremor and rotation are ignored.

Estimate the patient's level of sensorium along a continuum, from alert on the left to coma on the right.

(From Folstein MF, Folstein SE, and McHugh PR: Mini-mental state. J Psychiatric Res 12:189–198, 1975. Reprinted with permission.)

Nursing Diagnoses Commonly Associated with Mental Health Disorders

Altered thought processes

Anxiety

Impaired adjustment

Ineffective individual coping

Low self-esteem

Personal identity disturbance

Potential for violence (self-directed or directed at others)

Powerlessness

3 Assessment Techniques and Approach to the Clinical Setting

ASSESSMENT TECHNIQUES

The skills requisite for the physical examination are inspection, palpation, percussion, and auscultation. The skills are performed one at a time and in this order.

Inspection

Inspection is close careful scrutiny, first of the individual as a whole and then of each body system. Inspection begins the moment you first meet the individual and develop a "general survey." (Specific data to consider for the general survey are presented in the following chapter.) As you proceed through the examination, start the assessment of each body system with inspection.

Learn to use each person as his or her own control and compare the right and left sides of the body. The two sides are nearly symmetric. Inspection requires good lighting, adequate exposure, and occasional use of instruments (otoscope, ophthalmoscope, penlight, nasal and vaginal specula) to enlarge your view.

Palpation

Palpation follows and often confirms points you noted during inspection. Palpation applies your sense of touch to assess these factors: texture, temperature, moisture, organ location and size, as well as any swelling, vibration or pulsation, rigidity or spasticity, crepitation, presence of lumps or masses, and presence of tenderness or pain. Different parts of the hands are best suited for assessing different factors:

- Fingertips—Best for fine tactile discrimination, such as skin texture, swelling, pulsatility, and determining presence of lumps.
- A grasping action of the fingers— To detect the position, shape, and consistency of an organ or mass.
- The dorsa (backs) of hands and fingers—Best for determining temperature because the skin here is thinner than on the palms.
- Base of fingers (metacarpophalangeal joints) or ulnar surface of the hand—Vibration.

Your palpation technique should be slow and systematic. Warm your hands by kneading them together or holding them under warm water. Identify any tender areas, and palpate them last.

Start with light palpation to detect surface characteristics and accustom the person to being touched.

When deep palpation is needed (as for abdominal contents), intermittent pressure is better than one, long, continuous palpation. Avoid any situation in which continuous or deep palpation could cause internal injury or pain.

Bimanual palpation requires the use of both hands to envelop or capture certain body parts or organs, such as the kidneys, uterus, or adnexa, for more precise delimitation.

Percussion

Percussion is tapping the person's skin with short, sharp strokes in order to assess underlying structures. The strokes yield a palpable vibration and a characteristic sound that depicts the location, size, and density of the underlying organ.

The Stationary Hand. Hyperextend the middle finger of your nondominant hand (sometimes called the pleximeter) and place its distal portion firmly against the person's skin. Avoid the person's ribs and scapulae. Percussing over a bone yields no data because it always sounds "dull." Lift the rest of the stationary hand up off the person's skin (Fig. 3–1); otherwise, the resting hand will dampen off the produced vibrations, just as a drummer uses the hand to halt a drum roll.

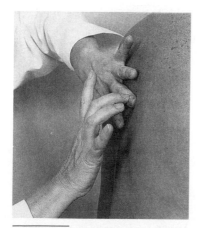

▶ Figure 3–1   Percussion

The Striking Hand. Use the middle finger of your dominant hand as the *striking* finger (sometimes called the plexor). Hold your forearm close to the skin surface with your upper arm and shoulder steady but not rigid. The action is all in the wrist and it *must* be relaxed.

Bounce your middle finger off the stationary one. Aim for just behind the nailbed. Flex the striking finger so that its tip, not the finger pad, makes contact. It hits directly at right angles to the stationary finger.

Percuss two times in this location using even, staccato blows. Lift the striking finger off quickly; a resting finger damps off vibrations. Then move to a new body location and repeat, keeping your technique even.

Table 3–1 describes five percussion notes heard in clinical practice and their expected location.

Auscultation

Auscultation is listening to sounds produced by the body, such as the heart, blood vessels, lungs, and abdomen, through a *stethoscope.*

Choose a stethoscope with two endpieces—a diaphragm and a bell. The *diaphragm* has a flat edge and is best for high-pitched sounds—breath, bowel, and normal heart sounds. Hold the diaphragm firmly against the person's skin, firm enough to leave a slight ring afterward.

The *bell* endpiece has a deep, hollow, cuplike shape. It is best for soft, low-pitched sounds, such as extra heart sounds or murmurs. Hold it lightly against the person's skin, just enough so it forms a perfect seal. Pressing harder causes the person's skin to act as a diaphragm, obliterating the low-pitched sounds.

SETTING

- The examination room—warm and comfortable, quiet, private, and well lit.
- When possible, stop any distracting noises.

Table 3–1 ▶ **Characteristics of Percussion Notes**

	Amplitude	Pitch	Quality
Resonant	Medium-loud	Low	Clear, hollow
Hyperresonant	Louder	Lower	Booming
Tympany	Loud	High	Musical and drumlike (like the kettle drum)
Dull	Soft	High	Muffled thud
Flat	Very soft	High	A dead stop of sound, absolute dullness

- Discourage interruptions.
- Lighting with natural daylight is best, although artificial light will suffice.
- Position a wall or stand lamp for high-intensity lighting.
- The examination table—position so that both sides are easily accessible and at a height at which you can stand without stooping.
- The table should be equipped to raise the person's head up to 45 degrees.
- A roll-up stool—for the sections of the examination for which you must be sitting.
- A bedside stand or table—to lay out all your equipment.

EQUIPMENT

Before the examination, have all your equipment within easy reach and laid out in an organized manner. These items are usually needed for a complete physical examination:

Platform scale with height attachment

Skinfold calipers

Sphygmomanometer

Stethoscope with bell and diaphragm endpieces

Thermometer

Flashlight or penlight

Otoscope/ophthalmoscope

Tuning fork

Nasal speculum (if a short, broad speculum is not included with the otoscope)

Tongue depressor

Pocket vision screener

Skin marking pen

Flexible tape measure and ruler marked in centimeters

Duration	Sample Location
Moderate	Over normal lung tissue
Longer	Normal over child's lung. In the adult, over lungs with abnormal amount of air as in emphysema
Sustained longest	Over air-filled viscus, e.g., the stomach, the intestine
Short	Relatively dense organ, as liver or spleen
Very short	When no air is present, over thigh muscles, bone, or over tumor

Reflex hammer

Sharp hammer (sterile needle or split-tongue blade)

Cotton balls

Bivalve vaginal speculum

Clean gloves

Materials for cytologic study

Lubricant

Guaiac test reagents

APPROACH TO THE CLINICAL SETTING

Preparation for a Complete Assessment

Most people, whether entering the hospital or receiving outpatient care, initially require a complete physical examination. Before you begin, ask the person to empty the bladder and save a urine specimen if needed.

Begin by measuring the person's height, weight, blood pressure, temperature, pulse, and respirations. If needed, measure visual acuity at this time using the Snellen eye chart.

Ask the person to change into an examining gown, leaving the underpants on. Unless your assistance is needed, leave the room as the person undresses.

As you re-enter the room, wash your hands in the person's presence. This indicates you are protective of this person and are starting fresh for him or her. Explain each step in the examination and how the person can cooperate. Encourage the person to ask questions. Keep your own movements slow, methodical, and deliberate.

As you proceed through the examination, avoid distractions and concentrate on one step at a time. The sequence of the steps may differ depending on the age of the person and your own preference; however, you should establish a system that works for you and stick to it to avoid omissions.

Organize the steps so the person does not change positions too often. Although proper exposure is necessary, use additional drapes to maintain the person's privacy and to prevent chilling.

(See Chapter 20 for the sequence of steps in the complete physical examination.)

The Ill Person

For the ill person in some distress, alter the position during the examination. A person with shortness of breath or ear pain, for example, may want to sit up, whereas a person with faintness or overwhelming fatigue may want to be supine. Initially, it may be necessary just to examine the body areas appropriate to the problem, collecting a *mini database*. You may return to finish a complete assessment after the initial distress is resolved.

Episodic or Problem-Centered Assessment

This is for a limited or short-term problem. Here, you collect a "mini" data base, smaller in scope than the complete assessment. It concerns mainly one problem, one cue complex, or one body system. It is used in all settings—hospital, primary care, or long-term care.

Follow-up Assessment

The status of any identified problems should be evaluated at regular and appropriate intervals. What change has occurred? Is the problem getting better or worse? What coping strategies are used? This type of assessment is used in all settings to follow up short-term or chronic health problems.

For more information on the preparation of infants, children, and older adults for the physical examination, see Jarvis: *Physical Examination and Health Assessment*, **pp. 173–177.**

4 The General Survey, Measurement, Vital Signs

THE GENERAL SURVEY

The general survey is an assessment of the whole person, covering the general health state and any obvious physical characteristics. Objective parameters are used to form the general assessment, but these apply to the whole person not just to one body system.

Begin building a general assessment from the moment you first encounter the person. What leaves an immediate impression?

As you proceed through the health history, the measurements, and the vital signs, note the following points that will add up to the general assessment: physical appearance, body structure, mobility, and behavior.

PHYSICAL APPEARANCE

Age—appears his or her stated age.

Sexual development—appropriate for gender and age.

Level of consciousness—alert and oriented, attends to questions, responds appropriately.

Skin color—Color tone is even, pigmentation varying with genetic background; skin is intact with no obvious lesions.

Facial features—symmetric with movement.

There are no signs of acute distress.

BODY STRUCTURE

Stature—The height appears within normal range for age and genetic heritage.

Nutrition—The weight appears within normal range for height and body build. Body fat distribution is even.

Symmetry—Body parts look equal bilaterally and are in relative proportion to each other.

Posture—Stands comfortably erect as appropriate for age.

Position—Sits comfortably in a chair or on the bed or examination table, arms relaxed at sides, head turned to examiner.

Body build, contour—Proportions are:

1. Arm span (fingertip to fingertip) equals height.

2. Body length from crown to pubis roughly equal to length from pubis to sole.

Obvious physical deformities—Note any congenital or acquired defects.

MOBILITY

Gait—Normally, the base is as wide as the shoulder width. Foot placement is accurate. The walk is smooth, even, and well-balanced; and associated movements, such as symmetric arm swing, are present.

Range of motion—Note full mobility for each joint and that movement is deliberate, accurate, smooth, and coordinated.

No involuntary movement is present.

BEHAVIOR

Facial expression—Maintains eye contact (unless there is a cultural taboo); expressions are appropriate to the situation, e.g., thoughtful, serious, or smiling.

Mood and affect—The person is comfortable and cooperative with the examiner and interacts pleasantly.

Speech—Articulation (the ability to form words) is clear and understandable. The stream of speech is fluent, with an even pace. The person conveys ideas clearly. Word choice is appropriate to culture and education. The person communicates in prevailing language easily by himself or herself or with an interpreter.

Dress—Clothing is appropriate to the climate, looks clean and fits the body, and is appropriate to the person's culture and age group.

Personal hygiene—Appears clean and groomed appropriately for his or her age, occupation, and socioeconomic group. Hair is groomed or brushed. Women's make-up is appropriate for age and culture.

MEASUREMENT

WEIGHT

Use a standardized *balance scale*. Instruct the person to remove his or her shoes and heavy outer clothing before standing on the scale. When a sequence of repeated weights is necessary, aim for approximately the same time of day and the same type of clothing worn each time. Record the weight in kilograms and in

pounds. The weight tables from the Metropolitan Life Insurance Company give a recommended range (Table 4–1).

Compare the person's weight with the previous health visit. A recent weight loss may be explained by dieting.

An unexplained weight loss may be a sign of a short-term illness (e.g., fever, infection, disease of the mouth or throat), or a chronic illness (endocrine disease, malignancy, mental health dysfunction).

A weight gain usually reflects overabundant caloric intake, unhealthy eating habits, or a sedentary lifestyle.

Obesity occasionally may be due to endocrine disorders, drug therapy (e.g., corticosteroids), or mental depression.

HEIGHT

Use the measuring pole on the balance scale. Align the extended headpiece with the top of the head. The person should be shoeless, standing straight, and looking straight ahead.

Arm Span or Total Arm Length

Measurement of arm span is useful for those situations in which height is difficult to measure, such as, in children with cerebral palsy or scoliosis or in aging persons with spinal curvature. Arm span, which is nearly equivalent to height, is sometimes used clinically instead of height.

Ask the person to hold the arms straight out from the sides of the body. Measure the distance from the tip of the middle finger on one hand to that on the other hand.

Skinfold Thickness

Skinfold thickness measurements provide an estimate of body fat stores or the extent of obesity or undernutrition. The triceps skinfold (TSF) is the site most commonly selected because of its easy accessibility and because standards and tech-

Table 4-1 ▶ Height and Weight Tables for Men and Women According to Frame, Ages 25-59

Height*		Weight**		
Feet	Inches	Small Frame	Medium Frame	Large Frame
Men				
5	2	128-134	131-134	138-150
5	3	130-136	133-143	140-153
5	4	132-138	135-145	142-156
5	5	134-140	137-148	144-160
5	6	136-142	139-151	146-164
5	7	138-145	142-154	149-168
5	8	140-148	145-157	152-172
5	9	142-151	148-160	155-176
5	10	144-154	151-163	158-180
5	11	146-157	154-166	161-184
6	0	149-160	157-170	164-188
6	1	152-164	160-174	168-192
6	2	155-168	164-178	172-197
6	3	158-172	167-182	176-202
6	4	162-176	171-187	181-207
Women				
4	10	102-111	109-121	118-131
4	11	103-113	111-123	120-134
5	0	104-115	113-126	122-137
5	1	106-118	115-129	125-140
5	2	108-121	118-132	128-143
5	3	111-124	121-135	131-147
5	4	114-127	124-138	134-151
5	5	117-130	127-141	137-155
5	6	120-133	130-144	140-159
5	7	123-136	133-147	143-163
5	8	126-139	136-150	146-167
5	9	129-142	139-153	149-179
5	10	132-145	142-156	152-173
5	11	135-148	145-159	155-176
6	0	138-151	148-162	158-179

* Shoes with 1 inch heels.
** Weight in pounds. Men: allow 5 lb of clothing. Women: allow 3 lb of clothing.
(Courtesy of Metropolitan Life Insurance Company, 1983.)

niques are most developed for this site. To measure triceps skinfold thickness:

1 ▶ Have the ambulatory person stand with arms hanging freely at the sides and back to the examiner.
2 ▶ Using the thumb and forefinger of your left hand, gently grasp a fold of skin and fat on the posterior aspect of the person's upper arm, midway between the acromion process of the scapula and the olecranon process (the tip of the elbow). Gently pull the skinfold away from the underlying muscle.
3 ▶ While grasping the skinfold, pick up the calipers with your right hand and depress the spring-loaded lever. Apply

caliper jaws horizontally to the fat fold. Release the lever of the calipers while holding the skinfold. Wait 3 seconds, then take a reading. Repeat three times and average the three skinfold measurements. (Fig. 4–1).

4 ▶ Record measurements to the nearest 5 mm (0.5 cm). Compare the person's measurements with standards by age and sex (see Tables 6–6 and 6–7 in Jarvis: *Physical Examination and Health Assessment,* **pp. 141–142).**

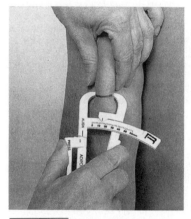

▶ Figure 4–1 Measuring triceps skinfold thickness

Triceps skinfold values that are 10 percent below or above standard are suggestive of undernutrition and overnutrition respectively. Conditions such as edema or subcutaneous emphysema may produce falsely high readings.

DEVELOPMENTAL CONSIDERATIONS

Infants and Children

Weight

Weigh an infant on a platform-type balance scale. To check calibration, set the weight at zero and observe the beam balance. Guard the baby so that he or she does not fall. Weigh to the nearest 10 g (½ oz) for infants and 100 g (¼ lb) for toddlers.

By age 2 or 3 years, use the upright scale. Leave underpants on the child. Some young children are fearful of the rickety standing platform and may prefer sitting on the infant scale. Use the upright scale with preschoolers and school-aged children, maintaining modesty with light clothing.

Length

Until age 2 years, measure the infant's body length supine using a horizontal measuring board. Hold the head in the midline. Because the infant normally has flexed legs, extend them momentarily by holding the knees together and pushing them down until the legs are flat on the table. Avoid using a tape measure along the infant's length because this is inaccurate.

By age 2 or 3 years, measure the child's height by standing the child against the pole on the platform scale or against a flat ruler taped to the wall. Encourage the child to stand straight and tall and to look straight ahead without tilting the head. The shoulders, buttocks, and heels should touch the wall. Hold a book or flat board on the child's head at a right angle to the wall. Mark just under the book or board, noting the measure to the nearest 1 mm (⅛ in).

Head Circumference

Measure the infant's head circumference at birth and at each well child visit up to age 2 years, then yearly up to age 6 years. Circle the tape around the head at the prominent frontal and occipital bones; the widest span is correct. Plot the measurement on standardized growth charts. Compare the infant's head size with that expected for age. A series of measurements is more valuable than a single figure to show the *rate* of head growth.

A newborn's head measures about 32–38 cm (average around 34 cm) and is about 2 cm larger than the chest circumference. The chest grows at a faster rate than the cranium; at some time between 6 months and 2 years, both measurements are about the same, and after age 2, the chest circumference is greater than the head circumference.

Measurement of the chest circumference is valuable as a comparison with the head circumference but is not necessarily valuable by itself. Circle the tape around the chest at the nipple line. It should be snug, but not too tight to leave a mark.

The Aging Adult

Weight

The aging person has more prominent bony landmarks than the younger adult. Body weight decreases during the 8th and 9th decades. This factor is more evident in males, perhaps because of greater muscle shrinkage. The distribution of fat also changes when persons are in their 80s and 90s. Subcutaneous fat is lost from the face and periphery (especially the forearms), whereas additional fat is deposited in the abdomen and hips.

Height

By the 8th and 9th decades, many people are shorter than they were in their 70s. This results from shortening of the spinal column due to thinning of the vertebral discs and shortening of the individual vertebrae, as well as postural changes of kyphosis and slight flexion in the knees and hips. Since long bones do not shorten with age, the overall body proportion appears different— a shorter trunk with relatively long extremities.

Kyphosis is an exaggerated posterior curvature of the thoracic spine (humpback). See Table 15–2, p. 175.

VITAL SIGNS

TEMPERATURE

The normal oral range in a resting person is 37°C (98.6°F), with a range of 35.8°F to 37.3°C (96.4°F to 99.1°F). The rectal temperature measures 0.4°C to 0.5°C (0.7°F to 1°F) higher. The normal temperature is influenced by:

• A diurnal cycle of 1°F to 1.5°F, with the trough occurring in the early morning hours and the peak occurring in late afternoon to early evening.
• The menstruation cycle in women. Progesterone secretion, occurring with ovulation at midcycle, causes a 0.5°F to 1.0°F rise in temperature that continues until menses.
• Exercise. Moderate to hard exercise increases body temperature.
• Age. Wider normal variations occur in the infant and young child due to less effective heat control mechanisms. In older adults, temperature is usually lower than in other age groups with a mean of 36.2°C (97.2°F).

Shake the *mercury-in-glass thermometer* down to 35.5°C (96°F) and place it at the base of the tongue in either of the posterior sublingual pockets, *not* in front of the tongue. Instruct the person to keep his or her lips closed. Leave in place 3–4 minutes if person is afebrile and up to 8 minutes if febrile. Wait 15 minutes if the person has just taken hot or iced liquids and 2 minutes if he or she has just smoked.

The *electronic thermometer* has the advantages of swift and accurate measurements (usually within 30 seconds) as well as safe, unbreakable, disposable probe covers. The instrument must be fully charged and correctly calibrated. Read the instructions carefully before use. Some types of electronic thermometers use the *same* probe for oral, rectal, or continuous temperatures, but other manufacturers supply different probes for different routes.

The *tympanic thermometer* is a noninvasive, nontraumatic device that is rapid and efficient. The probe tip is shaped like an otoscope. Gently place the covered probe tip in the person's ear canal. Do not force it and do not occlude the canal. Activate the device and read the temperature in 2 seconds.

PULSE

Using the pads of your first three fingers, palpate the radial pulse at the flexor aspect of the wrist laterally along the radius bone. Push until you feel the strongest pulsation. If the rhythm is regular, count the number of beats in 15 seconds and multiply by 4. If however, the rhythm is irregular, count for 1 full minute. As you begin the counting interval, start your count with "zero" for the first pulse felt. The second pulse felt is "one" and so on.

In the resting adult, the normal heart rate range is 60 to 100 beats per minute (bpm), although the well-conditioned althlete may have a resting rate as low as 50 bpm. The rate normally varies with age, being more rapid in infancy and childhood and more moderate during adult and older years. The rate also varies with sex; after puberty, females have a slightly faster rate than males.

RESPIRATIONS

Normally, a person's breathing is relaxed, regular, automatic, and silent. Since most people are unaware of their breathing, do not mention that you will be counting the respirations because sudden awareness may alter the normal pattern. Instead, maintain your position of counting the radial pulse and unobtrusively count the respirations. Count for 30 seconds if respirations are normal or for 1 full minute if you suspect an abnormality. Avoid the 15 second interval because the result can vary by a factor of $+$ or -4, which is significant with such a small number.

Respiratory rates are 10 to 20 breaths per minute for adults and are normally more rapid in infants and children. A fairly constant ratio of pulse rate to respiratory rate also exists, which is about $4:1$. Normally, both pulse and respiratory rates rise as a response to exercise or anxiety.

BLOOD PRESSURE

Blood pressure is the force of the blood pushing against the side of the vessel wall. The *systolic* pressure is the maximum pressure felt on the artery during left ventricular contraction, or systole. The *diastolic* pressure is the elastic recoil, or resting pressure that the blood constantly exerts between each contraction. The *pulse pressure* is the difference between the systolic and diastolic pressures and reflects the stroke volume.

The average blood pressure in young adults is 120/80 mmHg, although this varies normally with many factors, such as:

• Age. Normally, there is a gradual rise through childhood and into adult years (Fig. 4–2).
• Sex. Before puberty, there is no difference between males and females. After puberty, females usually show a lower blood pressure reading than their male counterparts. After menopause, blood pressure in females is higher than in male counterparts.
• Race. In the United States, a black adult's blood pressure is usually higher than whites of the same age. The incidence of hypertension is twice as high in blacks as in whites. The reasons for this difference are not understood fully but appear to be due to genetic heritage and environmental factors.
• Diurnal rhythm. There is a daily cycle of a peak and a trough: blood pressure climbs to a high in late afternoon or early evening and then declines to an early morning low.
• Weight. Blood pressure is higher in obese persons than in persons of

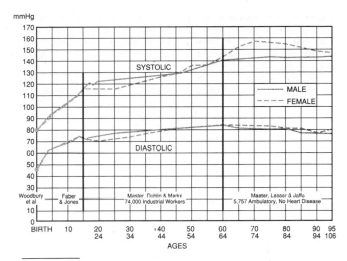

▶ Figure 4–2   Mean blood pressure readings in apparently healthy persons from birth to old age.

normal weight of the same age (including adolescents).

- Exercise: Increasing activity yields a proportionate increase in blood pressure. Within 5 minutes of terminating exercise, blood pressure normally returns to baseline.
- Emotions. Blood pressure momentarily rises with fear, anger, and pain as a result of stimulation of the sympathetic nervous system.
- Stress. Blood pressure is elevated in persons experiencing continual tension because of lifestyle, occupational stress, or life problems.

Blood pressure is measured using a stethoscope and a *sphygmomanometer* of either the mercury or aneroid type.

The cuff consists of an inflatable rubber bladder inside a cloth cover. The width of the rubber bladder should equal 40% of the circumference of the extremity used. The length of the bladder should equal 80% of this circumference.

The size is important; using a cuff that is too narrow yields a falsely high blood pressure. Match the appropriate size cuff to the person's arm size and shape and not to the person's age.

Arm Pressure. A comfortable, relaxed person yields a valid blood pressure. Many people are anxious at the beginning of an examination; if this is the case with the person being examined, retake the blood pressure later.

The person may be sitting or lying, with the bare arm supported at the heart level. Palpate the brachial artery, which is located just above the antecubital fossa medially. With the cuff deflated, center it about 2.5 cm (1 in.) above the brachial artery and wrap it evenly. Now palpate the brachial or the radial artery. Inflate the cuff until the artery pulsation is obliterated and then 20 to 30 mmHg beyond. This will avoid missing an *auscultatory gap* (i.e. sounds temporarily disappear), which is common with hypertension.

Place the stethoscope over the site of the brachial artery, making a light but airtight seal. Deflate the cuff slowly and evenly, about 2 mmHg per heartbeat. Note the points at which you hear the first appearance of sound, the muffling of sound, and the final disappearance of sound. These are phases I, IV, and V of *Korotkoff's sounds*.

In children, phase IV (muffling) is the more accurate measure of diastolic pressure, while in adults, phase V (the last audible sound) best indicates diastolic pressure. When a variance greater than 10–12 mmHg exists between phase IV and V, however, record *both* phases along with the systolic reading, e.g., 142/98/80. Clear communication is important because results significantly affect diagnosis and planning of care. Table 4–2 presents a list of common errors in blood pressure measurement.

If the person is known to have hypertension, is taking antihypertensive medications, or reports a history of fainting or syncope, take the blood pressure reading in three positions—lying down, sitting, and standing. Normally there may be a slight decrease (less than 10 mmHg) in systolic pressure when the position is changed from supine to standing.

Orthostatic hypotension, a drop in systolic pressure of more than 20 mmHg, may occur with a quick change to a standing position. It is due to abrupt peripheral vasodilation without a compensatory increase in cardiac output. Aging people have the greatest risk of this problem. It also occurs with prolonged bedrest, hypovolemia, and some drugs. Table 4–3 presents further information on hypotension and hypertension.

DEVELOPMENTAL CONSIDERATIONS

The aorta and major arteries tend to harden with age. As the heart pumps against a stiffer aorta, the systolic pressure increases, leading to a widened pulse pressure (See

---

Table 4–2 ▶ Common Sources of Error in Blood Pressure Measurement

Errors that produce a falsely *high* reading

▶ Failure to use the appropriate cuff size; a too narrow cuff gives a higher reading
▶ Wrapping the cuff too loosely or unevenly (cuff pressure must be exceedingly high to compress the brachial artery)
▶ Recording BP just after a meal, while person is smoking, or while person's bladder is distended
▶ Failure to have the mercury column vertical
▶ Deflating the cuff too slowly; this produces venous congestion in the extremity, which falsely elevates diastolic pressure

Errors that produce a falsely *low* reading

▶ Having the person's arm above the level of the heart (effect of hydrostatic pressure can give an error up to 10 mmHg in systolic and diastolic pressure)
▶ Failure to notice an auscultatory gap
▶ Diminished hearing acuity of the health care professional
▶ Stethoscope that is too small or too large, or has tubing that is too long
▶ Inability to hear feeble Korotkoff sounds

Errors that produce *either* falsely *high* or *low* readings

▶ Inaccurately calibrated manometer
▶ Defective equipment (valve, connections)
▶ Failure to have meniscus of mercury at eye level
▶ Performing the technique too quickly, with too little attention to details

(From Jarvis, C. M.: Assessing pulse, respiration, and blood pressure. In: Sorensen, K. C., and Luckmann, J.: Basic Nursing, A Pathophysiological Approach. 2nd ed. Philadelphia, W. B. Saunders, 1986, p. 545, with permission.)

Table 4-3 ▶ Abnormalities in Blood Pressure

HYPOTENSION

In normotensive adults: Below 95/60

In hypertensive adults: Below the person's average reading, but above 95/60

In children: Below expected value for age

Occurs With	Rationale
Acute myocardial infarction	Decreased cardiac output
Shock	Decreased cardiac output
Hemorrhage	Decrease in total blood volume
Vasodilation	Decrease in peripheral vascular resistance
Addison's disease (hypofunction of adrenal glands)	

Associated Symptoms and Signs

In conditions of decreased cardiac output, a low BP is accompanied by an increased pulse, dizziness, diaphoresis, confusion, and blurred vision. The skin feels cool and clammy because the superficial blood vessels constrict to shunt blood to the vital organs. An individual having an acute MI (myocardial infarction) may also complain of crushing substernal chest pain, high epigastric pain, and shoulder or jaw pain.

HYPERTENSION

In adults under 40:   >140/90

In adults over 40:   >160/95

In children: >95th percentile expected for age

(Diagnosis follows at least three separate elevated readings, not on one isolated high value.)

Essential or Primary Hypertension

This occurs from no known cause but is responsible for about 95 percent of cases of hypertension in adults.

Secondary Hypertension

This is due to a specific, often curable cause and occurs with:
Kidney disease
  Renal vascular disease
  Pyelonephritis
  Glomerulonephritis
  Renal failure
  Renal injury
  Renal tumor
Adrenal disorder
  Cushing's disease
  Pheochromocytoma (tumor of adrenal medulla)
  Hyperaldosteronism
Coarctation of the aorta
Central nervous system disorders
  Brain tumor
  Head injury
Medication side effect
  Pressor agents (epinephrine, isoproterenol, ephedrine)
  Corticosteroids
  Oral contraceptives
  Amphetamines
Volume overload ·

Fig. 4–2 for mean blood pressure readings in apparently healthy persons from birth to old age). With many older people, both the systolic and diastolic pressures increase, making it difficult to distinguish normal aging values from abnormal hypertension.

THE DOPPLER TECHNIQUE

The Doppler technique is used to locate peripheral pulse sites. For blood pressure measurement, the Doppler technique will augment Korotkoff's sounds when they are hard to hear with a stethoscope, such as those in infants with small arms and in obese persons in whom the sounds are muffled by layers of fat. Proper cuff placement is also difficult on the obese person's cone-shaped upper arm. In this situation, you can place the cuff on the more even forearm and hold the Doppler probe over the radial artery (Fig. 4–3). For either location, use this procedure:

- Apply coupling gel to the transducer probe.
- Turn Doppler on.
- Touch the probe to the skin, holding the probe perpendicular to the artery.

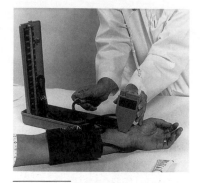

▶ Figure 4–3   Measuring BP using the Doppler technique

- A pulsatile whooshing sound indicates location of the artery. You may need to rotate the probe, but maintain contact with the skin. Do not push the probe too hard or you will wipe out the pulse.
- Inflate the cuff until the sounds disappear, then proceed another 20–30 mmHg beyond that point.
- Slowly deflate the cuff, noting the point at which the first whooshing sounds appear. This is the systolic pressure.
- A muffling of sounds indicates the diastolic pressure (phase IV of Korotkoff's sounds).

5 Skin, Hair, and Nails

The skin has two layers—the outer, highly-differentiated *epidermis* and the inner supportive *dermis* (Fig. 5-1). Beneath these layers is a third layer—the *subcutaneous* layer of adipose tissue.

The *sebaceous* glands produce a protective lipid, sebum, which is se-creted through the hair follicles. The *eccrine* glands are coiled tubules that open directly onto the skin surface and produce the sweat that helps reduce body temperature. The *apocrine* glands open into hair follicles and become active during puberty.

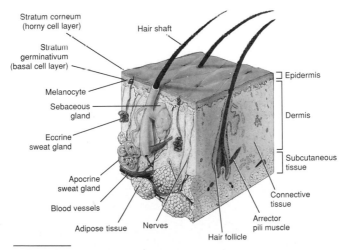

Stratum corneum (horny cell layer)
Stratum germinativum (basal cell layer)
Melanocyte
Sebaceous gland
Eccrine sweat gland
Apocrine sweat gland
Blood vessels
Adipose tissue
Nerves
Hair shaft
Epidermis
Dermis
Subcutaneous tissue
Connective tissue
Arrector pili muscle
Hair follicle

▶ Figure 5-1

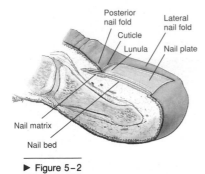

Posterior nail fold
Lateral nail fold
Cuticle
Lunula
Nail plate
Nail matrix
Nail bed

▶ Figure 5-2

The nails are hard plates of keratin on the dorsal edges of the fingers and toes (Fig. 5-2). The nail plate is clear with fine, longitudinal ridges that become prominent with older age. Nails take their pink color from the underlying nailbed of highly vascular epithelial cells.

TRANSCULTURAL CONSIDERATIONS

Melanin is responsible for the various colors and tones of skin among people from culturally diverse backgrounds. Melanin protects the skin against harmful ultraviolet rays, a genetic advantage accounting for the lower incidence of skin cancer among darkly pigmented black and Native American people.

The hair of black people varies widely in texture. It is very fragile and ranges from long and straight to short, spiraled, thick, and kinky. The hair and scalp have a natural tendency to be dry and require daily combing, gentle brushing, and the application of oil. By comparison, people of Asian backgrounds generally have straight, silky hair.

SUBJECTIVE DATA

Previous history of skin disease (allergies, hives, psoriasis, eczema)

Change in pigmentation

Change in mole (size or color)

Excessive dryness or moisture

Pruritus

Excessive bruising

Rash or lesion

Medications (any that cause allergic skin response, increased sunlight sensitivity)

Hair loss

Change in nails

Environmental or occupational hazards (sun exposure, toxic chemicals, insect bites)

Self-care behaviors (daily hygiene, use of soaps, cosmetics, chemicals)

OBJECTIVE DATA

Equipment Needed

Strong direct lighting (natural daylight is ideal to evaluate skin characteristics but is usually not available in the clinical area)

Small centimeter ruler

Penlight

METHOD OF EXAMINATION

NORMAL RANGE OF FINDINGS	ABNORMAL FINDINGS

SKIN
Inspect and Palpate

Color

General Pigmentation. The skin tone is consistent with genetic background and varies from pinkish tan to ruddy dark tan, or from light to dark brown, and may have yellow or olive overtones. Dark-skinned people normally have areas of lighter pigmentation on the palms, nailbeds, and lips.

General pigmentation is darker in sun-exposed areas. Common (benign) pigmentations also occur:

• Freckles (ephelides)—a small, flat increase of brown melanin pigment.
• Moles (pigmented nevi)—a proliferation of melanocytes, tan to brown color, flat or raised.
• Birthmarks—may be tan to brown color.

Advise anyone with moles or birthmarks to perform periodic skin self-examinations. Watch for danger signs listed here. Ask a family member to check any areas the person cannot see (e.g., the back).

Danger signs: Note the following in pigmented lesions and refer.

1 ▶ Sudden enlargement
2 ▶ Change in color
3 ▶ An irregular border with notching or a butterfly shape, or a previously flat mole becoming elevated
4 ▶ Variegated color, i.e., an irregular range of blue, red, white, mixed with brown or black
5 ▶ Clumping of pigment
6 ▶ Change in surface features (scaling, flaking, oozing)
7 ▶ Change in sensation (itching, tenderness)
8 ▶ Change in surrounding skin (redness, swelling)
9 ▶ Ulceration or bleeding in mole (late sign)

Widespread Color Change. Note any pallor (white), erythema (red), cyanosis (blue), and jaundice (yellow). In dark-skinned people, the amount of normal pigment may mask color changes. Lips and nailbeds may not always be accurate signs. The more reliable sites are those with the least pigmentation, such as under the tongue, the buccal mucosa, the palpebral conjunctiva, and the sclera. Table 5–1 on p. 39 presents specific clues to assessment.

NORMAL RANGE OF FINDINGS	ABNORMAL FINDINGS

Temperature

Use the backs (dorsa) of your hands and palpate bilaterally. The skin should be warm, and equal bilaterally. Hands and feet may be slightly cooler in a cool environment.

Hypothermia. Generalized coolness may be induced, such as in hypothermia used for surgery or high fever. Localized coolness is expected with an immobilized extremity, as when a limb is in a cast or with an IV infusion.

General hypothermia accompanies central circulatory disturbance, such as with shock. Localized hypothermia occurs in peripheral arterial insufficiency and in Raynaud's disease due to vasospasm.

Hyperthermia. Generalized hyperthermia occurs with an increased metabolic rate, such as in fever, or after heavy exercise. A localized area feels hyperthermic with trauma, infection, or sunburn.

Warm moist skin occurs with hyperthyroidism due to hypermetabolic state.

Moisture

Perspiration appears normally on the face, hands, axilla, and skin folds in response to activity, a warm environment, or anxiety. *Diaphoresis,* or profuse perspiration, accompanies an increased metabolic rate, such as occurs in heavy activity or fever.

Diaphoresis occurs with thyroxicosis and with stimulation of the nervous system with anxiety or pain.

Dehydration is evident in the oral mucous membranes. They look dry, and the lips looked parched and cracked. Be aware that dark skin may normally look dry and flaky, but this does not necessarily indicate systemic dehydration.

With extreme dryness the skin is fissured, resembling cracks in a desert.

Texture

Normal skin feels smooth and firm, with an even surface.

Hyperthyroidism—the skin feels smoother and softer, like velvet. Hypothyroidism—the skin feels rough, dry, and flaky.

Thickness

The epidermis is uniformly thin over most of the body, although thickened callus areas are normal on palms and soles. A callus is a circumscribed overgrowth of epidermis and is an adaptation to excessive pressure.

Very thin, shiny skin (atrophic) occurs with arterial insufficiency.

| NORMAL RANGE OF FINDINGS | ABNORMAL FINDINGS |

Edema

To check for edema, imprint your thumbs firmly against the ankle malleolus or the tibia. Normally, the skin surface stays smooth when you lift your thumbs. If your pressure leaves a dent in the skin, "pitting" edema is present. Its presence is graded on a 4-point scale: from 1+ for mild edema to 4+ for deep pitting edema. This scale is somewhat subjective; outcomes vary among examiners.

Edema masks normal skin color as well as obscures pathologic conditions such as jaundice or cyanosis because the fluid lies between the surface and the pigmented and vascular layers. It makes dark skin look lighter.

Edema is fluid accumulating in the intercellular spaces and is not normally present. Edema is most evident in dependent parts of the body (feet, ankles, and sacral areas), where the skin looks puffy and tight. Edema makes the hair follicles more prominent, so you note a pigskin or orange-peel look.

Unilateral edema—consider a local or peripheral cause.

Bilateral edema or edema that is generalized over the whole body (anasarca)—consider a central problem such as congestive heart failure or kidney failure.

Mobility and Turgor

Pinch up a large fold of skin on the anterior chest under the clavicle. Mobility is the skin's ease of rising, and turgor is its ability to return to place promptly when released.

Mobility is decreased when edema is present.

Poor turgor is evident in severe dehydration or extreme weight loss; the pinched skin recedes slowly or "tents" and stands by itself.

Hygiene

Skin should be clean and free of body odor.

Vascularity or Bruising

Cherry (senile) angiomas are small, punctate, slightly raised, bright red dots that commonly appear on the trunk in all adults over 30. They normally increase in size and number with aging.

Any bruising should be consistent with the expected trauma of life. There is normally no venous dilation or varicosity.

Document to presence of any tattoos (a permanent skin design from indelible pigment) on the person's chart. Advise the person that the use of tattoo needles and tattoo

Multiple bruises at different stages of healing and excessive bruises above the knees or elbows should raise concern about physical abuse.

Needle marks or tracks from IV injection of street drugs may be visible on the antecubital fossae or forearms, or on any available vein.

NORMAL RANGE OF FINDINGS	ABNORMAL FINDINGS

parlor equipment of doubtful sterility increases the risk of hepatitis.

Lesions

Note:

1 ► Color
2 ► Elevation: flat, raised, or pedunculated
3 ► Pattern or shape: The grouping or distinctness of each lesion, for example, annular, grouped, confluent, linear. The pattern may be characteristic of a certain disease.
4 ► Size, in centimeters: Use a ruler to measure. Avoid descriptions such as "quarter size," or "pea size."
5 ► Location and distribution on body. Is it generalized or localized to area of a specific irritant: around jewelry, watchband, around eyes?
6 ► Any exudate? Note its color or odor.

Lesions are traumatic or pathologic changes in previously normal structures. When a lesion develops on previously unaltered skin, it is primary. When a lesion changes over time, however, or changes due to a factor such as scratching or infection, it is secondary. Study Table 5-2, p. 41 for pattern, and Tables 5-3 and 5-4 pp. 42-45 for the characteristics of primary and secondary skin lesions.

HAIR

Inspect and Palpate

Color

Hair color comes from melanin production and may vary from pale blonde to total black. Graying begins as early as the third decade of life due to genetic factors.

Texture

Scalp hair may be fine or thick and may look straight, curly, or kinky. It should look shiny.

Note dull, course, or brittle scalp hair.

Lesions

The scalp should be clean and free of any lesions or pest inhabitants. Many people normally have seborrhea (dandruff) which is indicated by loose white flakes.

Distinguish dandruff from nits (eggs) of lice, which are oval, adherent to the hair shaft, and cause intense itching.

NORMAL RANGE OF FINDINGS	ABNORMAL FINDINGS

NAILS

Inspect and Palpate

Shape and Contour

The nail surface is normally slightly curved or flat, and the posterior and lateral nail folds are smooth and rounded. Nail edges are smooth, rounded, and clean, suggesting adequate self-care.

Spoon nails (concave curves) may occur with iron deficiency anemia.

Paronychia (inflammation of base of nail) occurs with trauma, infection.

Jagged nails, bitten to the quick, or traumatized nail folds from chronic nervous picking suggest nervous habits.

Chronically dirty nails suggest poor self-care or some occupations in which it is impossible to keep them clean.

View the index finger at its profile and note the angle of the nail base; it should be about 160 degrees. The nail base is firm to palpation. Curved nails are a variation of normal with a convex profile. They may look like clubbed nails but notice that the angle between nail base and nail is normal, i.e., 160 degrees or less.

Clubbing of nails occurs with congenital, chronic, cyanotic heart disease and with emphysema and chronic bronchitis.

In early clubbing, the angle straightens out to 180 degrees and the nail base feels spongy to palpation (see Fig. 9–7, p. 241 in Jarvis: *Physical Examination and Health Assessment*).

Consistency

The surface is smooth and regular, not brittle or splitting

Pits, transverse grooves, or lines may indicate a nutrient deficiency or may accompany acute illness in which nail growth is disturbed.

Nail thickness is uniform.

Nails are thickened and ridged with arterial insufficiency.

The nail is firmly adherent to the nailbed, and the nail base is firm to palpation.

A spongy nail base accompanies clubbing.

Color

The translucent nail plate shows a pink nailbed underneath.

Dark-skinned people may have brown-black pigmented areas or linear bands or streaks along the nail edge. All people normally may have white hairline linear markings from

Cyanosis or marked pallor.

Brown linear streaks are abnormal in light-skinned people and may indicate melanoma.

Splinter hemorrhages occur with subacute bacterial endocarditis;

NORMAL RANGE OF FINDINGS	ABNORMAL FINDINGS

trauma or picking at the cuticle. Note any abnormal marking in the nailbeds.

transverse ridges, or Beau's lines, occur with trauma.

Depress the nail edge to blanch and then release, noting the return of color. Normally, color return is instant or within a few seconds in a cold environment. This indicates the status of the peripheral circulation. A sluggish color return takes longer than 1 or 2 seconds.

Cyanotic nailbeds or sluggish color return: consider cardiovascular or respiratory dysfunction.

DEVELOPMENTAL CONSIDERATIONS

Infants

General Pigmentation. Black newborns initially have lighter toned skin than their parents. Their full melanotic color is evident in the nailbeds and scrotal folds.

The *Mongolian spot* is a common variation of hyperpigmentation in black, Native American, Latin, and Asian newborns due to deep dermal melanocytes. It is a blue-black to purple macular area usually found at the sacrum or buttocks. It gradually fades during the first year.

Adolescents

The increase in sebaceous gland activity creates increased oiliness and acne.

The Pregnant Female

Striae are jagged linear "stretch marks" of silver to pink color that appear during the second trimester on the abdomen, breasts, and sometimes on the thighs. They occur in one-half of all pregnancies and fade after delivery but do not disappear. Another skin change on the abdomen is the *linea nigra,* a brownish black line down the midline.

Chloasma is an irregular brown patch of hyperpigmentation on the face. It may occur with pregnancy

NORMAL RANGE OF FINDINGS   ABNORMAL FINDINGS

or in women taking oral contraceptive pills. Chloasma disappears after delivery or cessation of pills.

Vascular spiders occur in two-thirds of pregnancies in white women but less often in black women. These lesions have tiny red centers with radiating branches and occur on the face, neck, upper chest, and arms.

The Aging Adult

Skin Color and Pigmentation. *Senile lentigines* are commonly called liver spots and are small, flat, brown macules that appear following extensive sun exposure on the forearms and dorsa of the hands. They are not malignant and require no treatment.

Moisture. Dry skin (xerosis) is common. The skin itches and appears flaky and loose.

Texture. *Acrochordons,* or "skin tags," are overgrowths of normal skin that form a stalk and occur frequently on eyelids, cheeks and neck, and axillae and trunk.

Thickness. With aging, the skin looks as thin as parchment and subcutaneous fat diminishes. Thinner skin is evident over the dorsae of the hands, forearms, lower legs, feet and bony prominences.

Mobility and Turgor. The turgor is decreased (less elasticity) and the skin recedes slowly or "tents" and stands by itself.

Hair. Hair growth decreases, and the amount decreases in the axillae and pubic areas. After menopause, white women may develop bristly hairs on the chin or upper lip resulting from unopposed androgens.

In men, coarse terminal hairs develop in the ears, nose, and eyebrows, although the beard is unchanged. Male-pattern balding, or *alopecia*, is a genetic trait. It is

NORMAL RANGE OF FINDINGS	ABNORMAL FINDINGS
usually a gradual receding of the anterior hairline in a symmetric **W** shape. In men and women, scalp hair gradually turns gray because of a decrease in melanocyte function. **Nails.** Nail growth rate decreases and local injuries in the nail matrix may produce longitudinal ridges. The surface may be brittle or peeling and sometimes yellowed. Toenails also are thickened and may grow misshapen, almost grotesque. The thickening may be a process of aging or due to chronic peripheral vascular disease. For more information on assessment of skin, hair, and nails, see Jarvis: *Physical Examination and Health Assessment,* **pp. 224–273**.	Fungal infections are common in aging, with thickened, crumbling toenails and erythematous scaling on contiguous skin surfaces.

A B N O R M A L   F I N D I N G S

Table 5-1 ▶ Color Changes in Light and Dark Skin

ETIOLOGY	LIGHT SKIN	DARK SKIN
PALLOR		
Anemia—decreased Hct Shock—decreased perfusion vasoconstriction	Generalized pallor	Brown skin appears yellow-brown, dull; black skin appears ashen gray, dull. Skin loses its healthy glow. Check areas with least pigmentation, such as conjunctivae, mucous membranes.
Local arterial insufficiency	Marked localized pallor, e.g., lower extremities, especially when elevated	Ashen gray, dull; cool to palpation
Albinism—total absence of pigment melanin throughout the integument	Whitish pink	Tan, cream, white
Vitiligo—patchy depigmentation from destruction of melanocytes	Patchy milky white spots, often symmetry bilaterally	Same
CYANOSIS		
Increased amount of unoxygenated hemoglobin Central—chronic heart and lung disease cause arterial desaturation	Dusky blue	Dark but dull, lifeless. Only severe cyanosis is apparent in skin. Check conjunctivae, oral mucosa, nailbeds.
Peripheral—exposure to cold, anxiety	Nailbeds dusky	
ERYTHEMA		
Hyperemia—increased blood flow through engorged arterioles, such as in inflammation, fever, alcohol intake, blushing	Red, bright pink	Purplish tinge, but difficult to see. Palpate for increased warmth with inflammation, for taut skin, and hardening of deep tissues
Polycythemia—increased RBCs, capillary stasis	Ruddy blue in face, oral mucosa, conjunctivae, hands and feet	Well concealed by pigment. Check for redness in lips.
Carbon monoxide poisoning	Bright cherry red in face and upper torso	Cherry red color in nailbeds, lips, and oral mucosa
Venous statis—decreased blood flow from area, engorged venules	Dusky rubor of dependent extremities. A prelude to necrosis with pressure sore	Easily masked; use palpation for warmth of edema

Table 5–1 ► Color Changes in Light and Dark Skin *Continued*

ETIOLOGY	LIGHT SKIN	DARK SKIN
JAUNDICE		
Increased serum bilirubin, over 2 to 3 mg/100 ml due to liver inflammation or hemolytic disease such as after severe burns, some infections	Yellow in sclerae, hard palate, mucous membranes, then over skin	Check sclera for yellow near limbus. Do not mistake normal yellowish fatty deposits in the periphery under the eyelids for jaundice. Jaundice best noted in junction of hard and soft palate; also palms.
Carotenemia—increased serum carotene from ingestion of large amounts of carotene-rich foods	Yellow-orange in forehead, palms and soles, nasolabial folds, but no yellowing in sclerae or mucous membranes	Yellow-orange tinge in palms and soles
Uremia—renal failure causes retained urochrome pigments in the blood	Orange-green or gray overlying pallor of anemia. May also have ecchymoses and purpura	Easily masked by dark skin; rely on laboratory and clinical findings
BROWN-TAN		
Addison's disease— cortisol deficiency stimulates increased melanin production	Bronzed appearance, an "eternal tan," most apparent around nipples, perineum, genitalia, and pressure points (inner thighs, buttocks, elbows, axillae)	Easily masked by dark skin; rely on lab and clinical findings
Café au lait spots—due to increased melanin pigment in basal cell layer	Tan to light brown, irregularly shaped, oval patch with well-defined borders.	

Table 5–2 ▶ Common Shapes of Skin Lesions

ANNULAR, or circular, begins in center and spreads to periphery, e.g., ringworm, tinea versicolor, pityriasis rosea

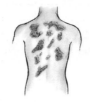

CONFLUENT, lesions run together, e.g., urticaria

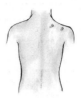

DISCRETE, distinct, individual lesions which remain separate

GROUPED, clusters of lesions, e.g., vesicles of contact dermatitis

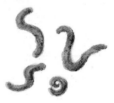

GYRATE, twisted, coiled spiral, snakelike

IRIS, or target, resembles iris of eye, concentric rings of lesions

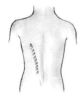

LINEAR, a scratch, streak, line, or stripe

POLYCYCLIC, annular lesions grow together

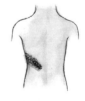

ZOSTERIFORM, linear arrangement along a nerve route, e.g., herpes zoster

Table 5–3 ▶ Primary Skin Lesions*

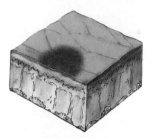

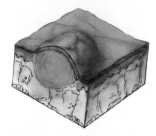

MACULE. Solely a color change, flat and circumscribed, less than 1 cm. Examples: freckles, flat nevi, hypopigmentation, petechiae, measles, scarlet fever

PATCH. Macules larger than 1 cm. Examples: mongolian spot, vitiligo, café au lait spot, chloasma, measles rash

PAPULE. Something you can feel, i.e., solid, elevated, circumscribed, less than 1 cm diameter. Examples: elevated nevus (mole), lichen planus, molluscum, wart (verrucae)

PLAQUE. Papules coalesce wider than 1 cm. A plateau-like, disc-shaped lesion. Examples: psoriasis, lichen planus

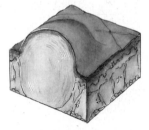

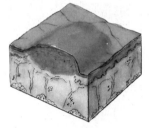

NODULE. Solid, elevated, hard or soft, larger than 1 cm. May extend deeper into dermis than papule. Examples: xanthoma, fibroma, intradermal nevi

TUMOR. Larger than a few centimeters in diameter, firm or soft, deeper into dermis; may be benign or malignant. Examples: lipoma, hemangioma

WHEAL. Superficial, raised, transient, and erythematous; slightly irregular shape due to edema (fluid held diffusely in the tissues). Examples: mosquito bite, allergic reaction, dermographism

URTICARIA (HIVES). Wheals coalesce to form extensive reaction, intensely pruritic.

Table 5–3 ► Primary Skin Lesions* *Continued*

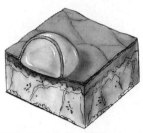

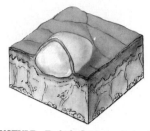

VESICLE. Elevated cavity containing free clear fluid, up to 1 cm. Examples: herpes simplex, early varicella (chicken pox), herpes zoster (shingles), contact dermatitis

PUSTULE. Turbid fluid (pus) in the cavity. Circumscribed and elevated. Examples: impetigo, acne

BULLA. Larger than 1 cm diameter; usually single-chambered (unilocular); superficial in epidermis, it is thin walled, so it ruptures easily. Examples: friction blister, pemphigus, burns, contact dermatitis

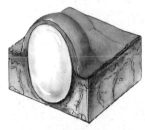

CYST. Encapsulated, fluid-filled cavity in dermis or subcutaneous layer, tensely elevating skin. Examples: sebaceous cyst, wen

* The immediate result of a specific causative factor; primary lesions develop on previously unaltered skin.

Table 5–4 ▶ Secondary Skin Lesions*

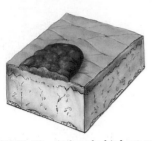

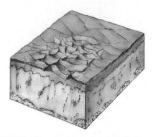

CRUST. The thickened, dried-out exudate left when vesicles/pustules burst or dry up. Color can be red-brown, honey, or yellow, depending on the fluid's ingredients (blood, serum, pus). Example: impetigo (dry, honey colored), weeping eczematous dermatitis, scab following abrasion

SCALE. Compact, desiccated flakes of skin, dry or greasy, silvery or white, from shedding of dead excess keratin cells. Examples: following drug reaction (laminated sheets), psoriasis (silver, micalike), seborrheic dermatitis (yellow, greasy), eczema, (large, adherent, laminated), dry skin

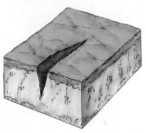

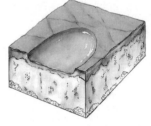

FISSURE. Linear crack with abrupt edges, extends into dermis, dry or moist. Examples: Cheilosis—at corners of mouth due to excess moisture; athlete's foot

EROSION. Scooped out but shallow depression. Superficial; epidermis lost; moist but no bleeding; heals without scar because erosion does not extend into dermis

* Resulting from a change in a primary lesion due to the passage of time; an evolutionary change.

Note: Combinations of primary and secondary lesions may coexist in the same person. Such combined designations may be termed papulosquamous, maculopapular, vesiculopustular, or papulovesicular.

Table 5–4 ▶ Secondary Skin Lesions* *Continued*

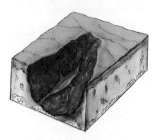

ULCER. Deeper depression extending into dermis, irregular shape; may bleed; leaves scar when heals. Examples: stasis ulcer, pressure sore, chancre

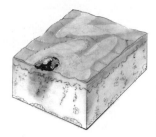

EXCORIATION. Self-inflicted abrasion; superficial; sometimes crusted; scratches from intense itching. Examples: insect bites, scabies, dermatitis, varicella

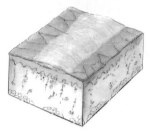

SCAR. After a skin lesion is repaired, normal tissue is lost and replaced with connective tissue (collagen). This is a permanent fibrotic change. Examples: healed area of surgery or injury, acne

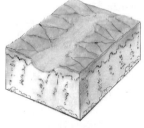

ATROPHIC SCAR. Resulting skin level depressed with loss of tissue; a thinning of the epidermis. Example: striae

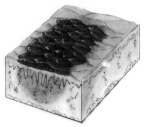

LICHENIFICATION. Prolonged intense scratching eventually thickens the skin and produces tightly packed sets of papules; looks like surface of moss (or lichen).

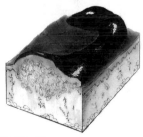

KELOID. Hypertrophic scar. The resulting skin level is elevated by excess scar tissue, which is invasive beyond the site of original injury. May increase long after healing occurs. Looks smooth, rubbery, "clawlike," and has a higher incidence among blacks.

☑ SUMMARY CHECKLIST

1 ▶ Inspect the skin for:
Color
General pigmentation
Areas of hypopigmentation or hyperpigmentation
Abnormal color changes
2 ▶ Palpate the skin for:
Temperature
Moisture
Texture
Thickness
Edema
Mobility and turgor
Hygiene
Vascularity or bruising

3 ▶ Note any lesions:
Color
Shape and configuration
Size
Location and distribution on body
4 ▶ Inspect and palpate the hair for:
Texture
Distribution
Any scalp lesions
5 ▶ Inspect and palpate the nails for:
Shape and contour
Consistency
Color

Nursing Diagnoses Commonly Associated with Skin, Hair, Nails Disorders

Impaired skin integrity

Fluid volume deficit

Self-care deficit: bathing/hygiene

Pain

Ineffective thermoregulation

Infection, potential for

Knowledge deficit

Body Image disturbance

Self-esteem disturbance

6 Head and Neck

The head and neck have a rich supply of lymph nodes (Fig. 6-1). The nodes are small oval clusters of lymphatic tissue. They filter the lymph and engulf pathogens, preventing potentially harmful substances from entering the circulation.

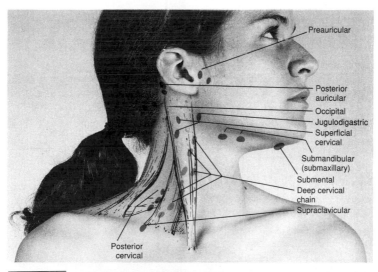

▶ Figure 6-1 Lymph nodes of the head and neck

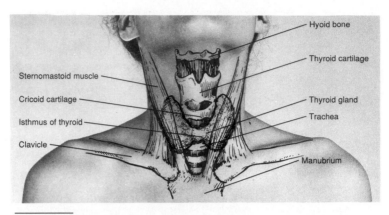

▶ Figure 6–2   Landmarks and structures in the neck

The neck contains many structures lying in close proximity (Fig. 6–2). The major neck muscles are the *sternomastoid* and the *trapezius* on the upper back. The carotid artery and internal jugular vein lie beneath the sternomastoid muscle. (Assessment of the neck vessels is discussed in Chapter 12.) The *thyroid gland* straddles the trachea and its two lobes each curve posteriorly between the trachea and sternomastoid muscle.

SUBJECTIVE DATA

Headache
Head injury
Dizziness

Neck pain
Limitation of motion
Lumps or swelling

OBJECTIVE DATA

METHOD OF EXAMINATION

NORMAL RANGE OF FINDINGS	ABNORMAL FINDINGS
THE HEAD **Inspect and Palpate the Skull** *Normocephalic* is a round, symmetric skull appropriately related to body size	Microcephaly, abnormally small head; macrocephaly, abnormally large head, e.g., hydrocephaly;

NORMAL RANGE OF FINDINGS	ABNORMAL FINDINGS
	and acromegaly (See Table 10–1, p. 301 in Jarvis: *Physical Examination and Health Assessment*).
The skull normally feels symmetrical and smooth. The cranial bones with normal protrusions are the forehead, the lateral edge of each parietal bone, the occipital bone, and the mastoid process behind each ear. There is no tenderness to palpation.	Note lumps, depressions, or abnormal protrusions.
Palpate the temporal artery above the zygomatic (cheek) bone between the eye and top of the ear.	
Palpate the temporomandibular joints located anterior to each ear as the person opens the mouth and note normally smooth movement with no limitation or tenderness.	Crepitation, limited range of motion, or tenderness.

Inspect the face

Note the facial expression and its appropriateness to behavior or reported mood. Anxiety is common in the hospitalized or ill person.	Hostility or embarrassment. Tense, rigid muscles may indicate anxiety or pain; a flat affect may indicate depression.
Note symmetry of eyebrows, palpebral fissures, nasolabial folds, and sides of the mouth. Note any abnormal facial structures (coarse facial features, exophthalmos, changes in skin color of pigmentation), or any abnormal swelling. Also note any involuntary movements (tics) in the facial muscles. Normally there are none.	Marked asymmetry with central brain lesion (e.g., cerebrovascular accident) or with peripheral cranial nerve VII damage (Bell's palsy) (See Table 10–5, pp. 305–307 in Jarvis: *Physical Examination and Health Assessment*).
	Edema in the face is noted first around the eyes (periorbital) and the cheeks where the subcutaneous tissue is relatively loose.
	Note grinding of jaws, tics, fasciculation, or excessive blinking.

THE NECK

Inspect and Palpate the Neck

Symmetry

Head position is in the midline; accessory neck muscles are symmetric.	Head tilt occurs with muscle spasm.
	Rigid head and neck occurs with arthritis.

NORMAL RANGE OF FINDINGS	ABNORMAL FINDINGS

Range of Motion

Note any limitation of movement. Ask the person to touch the chin to the chest, turn the head to the right and left, try to touch each ear to the shoulder (without elevating shoulders), and to extend the head backward. When the neck is supple, motion is smooth and controlled.

Note pain at any particular movement.

Note ratchety movement or limitation of movement that may be due to cervical arthritis or inflammation of neck muscles. With arthritis, the neck is rigid and the person turns at the shoulders rather than the neck.

Lymph Nodes

Using a gentle circular motion of your fingerpads and beginning with the preauricular lymph nodes in front of the ear, palpate the 10 groups of lymph nodes in a routine order. Be systematic and thorough. Use gentle pressure because strong pressure could push the nodes into the neck muscles. It is usually most efficient to palpate with both hands, comparing the two sides symmetrically.

If any nodes are palpable, note their location, size, shape, delimitation (discrete or matted together), mobility, consistency, and tenderness. Cervical nodes often are palpable in healthy persons, although palpability decreases with age. Normal nodes feel movable, discrete, soft, and nontender.

If nodes are enlarged or tender, check the area they drain for the source of the problem. Look *proximal* (upstream) to the location of the node; for example, those nodes in the upper cervical or submandibular areas often relate to inflammation or a neoplasm in the head and neck. Follow up on or refer your findings. An enlarged lymph node, particularly when you cannot find the source of the problem, deserves attention.

Lymphadenopathy—enlargement of the lymph nodes due to infection, allergy, or neoplasm.

The following are commonly associated with lymphadenopathy but are not definitive in all circumstances.

- Acute infection—nodes are bilateral, enlarged, warm, tender, and firm but freely moveable.
- Chronic inflammation, e.g., in tuberculosis the nodes are clumped.
- Cancerous nodes are hard, unilateral, nontender and fixed.
- Nodes with asymptomatic human immunodeficiency virus (HIV) infection are firm but not hard, and are nontender and mobile.
- An enlarged supraclavicular node may indicate a neoplasm in the thorax or abdomen.

NORMAL RANGE OF FINDINGS	ABNORMAL FINDINGS

Thyroid Gland

Position a standing lamp to shine tangentially across the neck to highlight any possible swelling. Supply the person with a glass of water and first inspect the neck as the person takes a sip and swallows. Thyroid tissue moves up with a swallow.

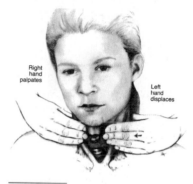

Right hand palpates

Left hand displaces

▶ Figure 6-3

To palpate the thyroid, move behind the person (Fig. 6-3). Ask the person to sit up very straight, then to bend the head slightly forward and to the right. This will relax the neck muscles. Use the fingers of your left hand to push the trachea slightly to the right.

Curve your right fingers between the trachea and the sternomastoid muscle, retracting it slightly, and ask the person to take a sip of water. The thyroid moves up under your fingers with the trachea and larynx as the person swallows. Reverse the procedure for the left side.

Usually you cannot palpate a normal adult thyroid. If the person has a long, thin neck, you sometimes will feel the thyroid isthmus over the tracheal rings. The lateral lobes usually are not palpable; check them for enlargement, consistency, symmetry, and the presence of nodules.

Abnormalities include enlarged lobes that are easily palpated before swallowing or are tender to palpation, or the presence of nodules or lumps. See Table 10-2, pp. 302-303 in Jarvis: *Physical Examination and Health Assessment.*

NORMAL RANGE OF FINDINGS	ABNORMAL FINDINGS

DEVELOPMENTAL CONSIDERATIONS

Infants and Children

An infant's head size is measured with measuring tape at each visit up to age 2. (Measurement of head circumference is presented in detail in Chapter 4).

Microcephalic—head circumference below norms for age.

Macrocephalic—an enlarged head for age or rapidly increasing in size. This may be due to hydrocephalus (increased cerebrospinal fluid).

Gently palpate the skull and fontanels while the infant is calm and in a somewhat sitting position (crying, lying down, or vomiting may cause the anterior fontanel to look full and bulging). The skull should feel smooth and fused except at the fontanels. The fontanels feel firm, slightly concave, and well defined against the edges of the cranial bones. You may see slight arterial pulsations in the anterior fontanel.

The posterior fontanel may not be palpable at birth. If it is, it measures 1 cm and closes by 1 to 2 months. The anterior fontanel may be small at birth and enlarge to 2.5 cm by 2.5 cm. A large diameter of 4 to 5 cm occasionally may be normal under 6 months.

The anterior fontanel closes between 9 months and 2 years. Early closure may be insignificant if head growth proceeds normally.

During infancy, cervical lymph nodes are not normally palpable, but a child's lymph nodes are—they feel more prominent than an adult's until puberty when lymphoid tissue begins to atrophy. Palpable nodes less than 3 mm are normal. They may be up to 1 cm in size in the cervical and inguinal areas but are discrete, move easily, and are nontender. Children have a higher incidence of infection, so you will expect a greater incidence of inflammatory adenopathy. There should be no other mass in the neck.

A true tense or bulging fontanel occurs with acute increased intracranial pressure.

Depressed and sunken fontanels occur with dehydration or malnutrition.

Marked pulsations occur with increased intracranial pressure.

Delayed closure or larger than normal fontanels occurs with hydrocephalus, Down syndrome, hypothyroidism, or rickets.

A small fontanel is a sign of microcephaly, as is early closure.

Cervical nodes larger than 1 cm are considered enlarged.

Thyroglossal duct cyst—cystic lymph node high up in the midline, freely movable, and rises up when swallowing.

Supraclavicular nodes enlarge with Hodgkin's disease.

NORMAL RANGE OF FINDINGS	ABNORMAL FINDINGS

The Pregnant Female

The thyroid gland may be normally palpable during pregnancy due to hyperplasia of the tissue and increased vascularity.

The Aging Adult

In some aging adults a mild rhythmic tremor of the head may be normal. *Senile tremors* are benign and include head nodding (as if saying yes or no) and tongue protrusion.

If some teeth have been lost, the lower face looks unusually small, with the mouth sunken in.

The neck may show an increased cervical concave curve when the head and jaw are extended forward to compensate for kyphosis of the spine. During the examination, direct the aging person to perform range of motion slowly; he or she may experience dizziness with side movements.

For more information on assessment of the head and neck, see Jarvis: *Physical Examination and Health Assessment*, pp. 276–307.

☑ SUMMARY CHECKLIST

1 ▶ Inspect and palpate the skull.
   General size and contour
   Note any deformities, lumps, tenderness
   Palpate temporal artery, temporomandibular joint
2 ▶ Inspect the face.
   Facial expression
   Symmetry of movement (cranial nerve VII)
   Any voluntary movements, edema, lesions
3 ▶ Inspect and palpate the neck.
   Active range of motion
   Enlargement of lymph nodes, thyroid gland

Nursing Diagnoses Commonly Associated with Head and Neck Disorders

Body image disturbance

Impaired swallowing

Impaired physical mobility

Pain

7 Eyes

ANATOMY

The eye is the sensory organ of vision. The eyelids protect the eye from injury, strong light, and dust (Fig. 7-1). The *palpebral fissure* is the open space between the eyelids.

The exposed part of the eye has a transparent protective covering, the *conjunctiva*. The *cornea* covers and protects the iris and pupil.

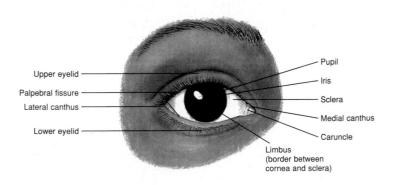

Upper eyelid

Palpebral fissure

Lateral canthus

Lower eyelid

Pupil

Iris

Sclera

Medial canthus

Caruncle

Limbus
(border between
cornea and sclera)

▶ Figure 7–1   External eye structures

The eye is a sphere composed of three concentric coats: (1) the outer fibrous *sclera,* (2) the middle vascular *choroid,* and (3) the inner nervous *retina* (Fig. 7–2). Inside the retina is the transparent vitreous body.

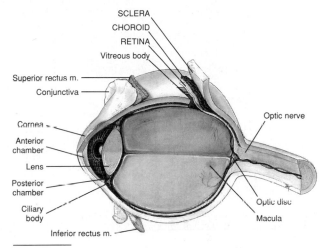

SCLERA
CHOROID
RETINA
Vitreous body
Superior rectus m.
Conjunctiva
Cornea
Anterior chamber
Lens
Posterior chamber
Ciliary body
Inferior rectus m.
Optic nerve
Optic disc
Macula

▶ Figure 7–2   Internal eye structures

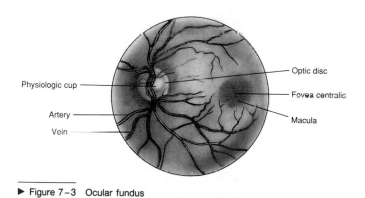

Physiologic cup
Artery
Vein
Optic disc
Fovea centralis
Macula

▶ Figure 7–3   Ocular fundus

The retina is the visual receptive layer of the eye in which light waves are changed into nerve impulses. The ocular fundus is the area of retina visible through the ophthalmoscope (Fig. 7–3).

The *optic disc* is the area in which fibers from the retina converge to form the optic nerve. The *macula* is the area of sharpest vision.

TRANSCULTURAL CONSIDERATIONS

 Racial differences are evident in the palpebral fissures. Persons of Asian origin are often identified by their characteristic eyes, whereas, the presence of narrowed palpebral fissures in non-Asian individuals may be diagnostic of a serious congenital anomaly, *Down syndrome.*

Individuals with darker irides have darker retinas behind them. Individuals with light retinas generally have better night vision but can suffer discomfort in an environment that has too much light.

S U B J E C T I V E   D A T A

Vision difficulty (decreased acuity, blurring, blind spots)

Pain

Strabismus, diplopia

Redness, swelling

Watering, discharge

Past history of ocular problems

Glaucoma

Does the person wear glasses or contact lenses

Self-care behaviors (vision last tested, method of care for contacts or glasses, efforts to protect eyes)

O B J E C T I V E   D A T A

Equipment Needed

Snellen eye chart

Hand-held visual screener

Opaque card or occluder

Penlight

Ophthalmoscope

Preparation

Position the person sitting up with his or her head at your eye level.

METHOD OF EXAMINATION

NORMAL RANGE OF FINDINGS	ABNORMAL FINDINGS
CENTRAL VISUAL ACUITY **Test visual acuity** **Snellen Eye Chart.** Position the person on a mark exactly 20 feet from the chart. Shield one eye at a time during the test. If the person wears glasses or contact lenses, leave them	

NORMAL RANGE OF FINDINGS

on. Ask the person to read through the chart to the smallest line of letters possible.

Record the result using the numeric fraction at the end of the last successful line read. Indicate whether or not the person missed any letters or if corrective lenses were worn, e.g., "O.D.* 20/30—1, with glasses."

Normal visual acuity is 20/20. The top number (numerator) indicates the distance the person is standing from the chart while the denominator gives the distance at which a normal eye can read a particular line.

Near Vision. For people over 40 years of age or for those who report increasing difficulty reading, test near vision using a hand-held vision screener with various sizes of print (e.g., a Jaeger card). Hold the card in good light about 35 cm (14 in) from the eye. Test each eye separately with glasses on. A normal result is "14/14" in each eye, read without hesitancy and without moving the card closer or farther away.

VISUAL FIELDS

Test Visual Fields

Confrontation Test. Position yourself at eye level with the person and about 2 feet away. Direct the person to cover one eye with an opaque card and to look straight at you with the other eye. Hold a pencil or your finger midline between you and the other person and slowly advance it in from the periphery in several directions (upward, downward, temporally, nasally).

ABNORMAL FINDINGS

Hesitancy, squinting, leaning forward, misreading letters.

The larger the denominator, the poorer the vision. If vision is poorer than 20/30, refer the person to an ophthalmologist or optometrist. Impaired vision may be due to refractive error, opacity in the media (cornea, lens, vitreous), or disorder in the retina or optic pathway.

Presbyopia, the decrease in power of accommodation with aging, is suggested when the card is moved farther away.

---

* O.D., oculus dexter, or right eye.

NORMAL RANGE OF FINDINGS	ABNORMAL FINDINGS

Ask the person to say "Now" as the object is first seen; this should be just as you see the object also.

If the person is unable to see the object as examiner does, the test suggests peripheral field loss. Refer the person for more precise testing using a tangent screen.

EXTRAOCULAR MUSCLE FUNCTION

Inspect Extraocular Muscle Function

Diagnostic Positions Test. Leading the eyes through the six *cardinal positions of gaze* will elicit any muscle weakness during movement. Ask the person to hold the head steady and follow the movement of your finger, pen, or penlight only with the eyes. Hold the object back about 12 inches so the person can focus on it comfortably and move it to each of the six positions, hold it momentarily, then back to center. Progress clockwise (Fig. 7–4). A normal response is parallel tracking of the object with both eyes.

Eye movement is not parallel. Failure to follow in a certain direction indicates weakness of an extraocular muscle (EOM) or dysfunction of the cranial nerve that innervates it.

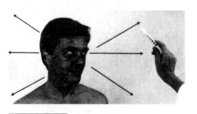

▶ Figure 7–4

In addition to parallel movement note any *nystagmus*, a fine oscillating movement best seen around the iris. Mild nystagmus at extreme lateral gaze is normal; nystagmus at any other position is not. Finally, note that the upper eyelid continues to overlap the superior part of the iris, even during downward movement. You should not see a white

Nystagmus

NORMAL RANGE OF FINDINGS	ABNORMAL FINDINGS

rim of sclera between the lid and the iris. If noted, this is referred to as "lid lag."

Lid lag occurs with hyperthyroidism.

EXTERNAL OCULAR STRUCTURES

Inspect External Structures

General. Note the person's ability to move around the room with vision functioning well enough to avoid obstacles and respond to your directions. The facial expression is relaxed with adequate vision.

Groping with hands.

Squinting or craning forward.

Eyebrows. Normally the eyebrows are present bilaterally, move symmetrically as the facial expression changes, and have no scaling or lesions.

Absent lateral third of eyebrows with hypothyroidism.
Unequal or absent movement with nerve damage.
Scaling with seborrhea.

Eyelids and Lashes. The upper lids normally overlap the superior part of the iris and approximate completely when closed. The skin is intact without redness, swelling, discharge, or lesions.

The palpebral fissures are horizontal in non-Asians, whereas palpebral fissures of Asians normally have an upward slant.

The eyelashes are evenly distributed along the lid margins and curve outward.

Lid lag with hyperthyroidism.
Incomplete closure creates risk for corneal damage.
Ptosis, drooping of upper lid.
Periorbital edema, lesions.

Ectropion and entropion (see Table 7–2, pages 67–68).

Eyeballs. The eyeballs are aligned normally with no protrusion or sunken appearance. Blacks may normally have a slight protrusion of the eyeball beyond the supraorbital ridge.

Exophthalmos, protruding eyes (see Table 7–2) and enophthalmos, sunken eyes.

Conjunctiva and Sclera. Ask the person to look up. Using your thumbs, slide the lower lids down along the bony orbital rim. Take care not to push against the eyeball. Inspect the exposed area. The eyeball looks moist and glossy. Numerous small blood vessels normally show through the transparent conjunctiva. Otherwise, the conjunctivae are clear and show the normal color of the structure below—pink

General reddening (injected) (see Table 7–2).
Cyanosis of the lower lids.
Pallor near the outer canthus of the lower lid may indicate

NORMAL RANGE OF FINDINGS	ABNORMAL FINDINGS

over the lower lids and white over the sclera. Note any color change, swelling, or lesions.

Blacks occasionally have a gray-blue or "muddy" color to the sclera. Dark-skinned people may have small brown macules (like freckles) on the sclera which should not be confused with foreign bodies or petechiae. Blacks may have yellowish fatty deposits beneath the lids away from the cornea. Do not confuse these yellow spots with the overall scleral yellowing that accompanies jaundice.

anemia (the inner canthus normally contains less pigment).

Scleral icterus is a yellowing of the sclera extending up to the cornea and indicating jaundice.

Tenderness, foreign body, discharge, or lesions.

ANTERIOR EYEBALL STRUCTURES

Inspect Anterior Eyeball Structures

Cornea and Lens. Shine a light from the side across the cornea and check for smoothness and clarity. There should be no opacities (cloudiness) in the cornea, anterior chamber, or in the lens behind the pupil. Do not confuse *arcus senilis* with an opacity. This is a normal finding in aging persons and is described on page 65.

A corneal abrasion causes irregular ridges in reflected light, usually visible only with fluorescein stain.

Iris and Pupils. The iris normally has a round regular shape and even coloration. Normally the pupils appear round, regular, and of equal size in 2both eyes. In the adult, resting size is from 3 to 5 mm. A small number of people (5 percent) have pupils of two different sizes, a condition called *anisocoria*.

To test the **pupillary light reflex,** darken the room and ask the person to gaze into the distance. (This dilates the pupils.) Advance a light in from the side* and note the re-

Irregular shape.

Unequally-sized pupils call for consideration of a central nervous system injury.

Dilated pupils.
Dilated and fixed pupils.
Constricted pupils.
Unequal or no response to light (see Table 7–3, pp. 68–69).

---

* Always advance the light in from the *side* to test the light reflex. If you advance from the front, the pupils will constrict to accommodate for near vision. Thus, you do not know what the pure response to the light would have been.

NORMAL RANGE OF FINDINGS

ABNORMAL FINDINGS

sponse. Normally you will see (1) constriction of the same-sided pupil (a *direct light reflex*) and (2) simultaneous constriction of the other pupil (a *consensual light reflex*).

Test for **accommodation** by asking the person to focus on a distant object. This process dilates the pupils. Then have the person shift the gaze to a near object, such as your finger held about 7 to 8 cm (3 in) from the nose. A normal response includes (1) pupillary constriction and (2) convergence of the axes of the eyes.

Record the normal response to all these maneuvers as PERRLA, or *Pupils Equal, Round, React to Light* and *Accommodation.*

Absence of constriction or convergence.
Asymmetric response.

THE OCULAR FUNDUS

Inspect the Ocular Fundus

Darken the room to help dilate the pupils. Remove eyeglasses from yourself or the other person; they obstruct close movement, and you can compensate for their correction by using the diopter setting. Contact lenses may be left in.

Select the large, round aperture with the white light for routine examination. If the pupils are small, use the smaller white light.

Tell the person, "Please keep looking at that light switch (or mark) on the wall across the room, even though my head will get in the way." Staring at a distant, fixed object helps dilate the pupils and hold the retinal structures still.

Match sides with the person: that is, hold the ophthalmoscope in your *right* hand up to your *right* eye to view the person's *right* eye. You must do this to avoid bumping noses during the procedure. Place your free hand on the person's shoulder or forehead.

Systematically inspect the structures in the ocular fundus: (1) optic disc, (2) retinal vessels, (3) general

NORMAL RANGE OF FINDINGS	ABNORMAL FINDINGS

background, and (4) macula (see Fig. 7–3). (Note the illustration shows a large area of the fundus. Your actual view through the ophthalmoscope is much smaller, slightly larger than 1 disc diameter.)

Optic Disc. The most prominent landmark is the optic disc, located on the nasal side of the retina. Explore these characteristics:

1 ▶ Color—Creamy yellow-orange to pink.

Pallor. Hyperemia.

2 ▶ Shape—Round or oval.

Irregular.

3 ▶ Margins—Distinct and sharply demarcated, though the nasal edge may be slightly fuzzy.

Blurred margins.

4 ▶ Cup-disc ratio—Distinctness varies. When visible, cup is a brighter yellow-white than rest of the disc. Its width is not more than one-half the disc diameter.

Cup extending to the disc border (see Table 11–11, pp. 358–359, in Jarvis: *Physical Examination and Health Assessment*).

Retinal Vessels. Follow a paired artery and vein out to the periphery in the four quadrants (See Fig. 7–3), noting these points:

1 ▶ Number—A paired artery and vein pass to each quadrant. Vessels look straighter at the nasal side.

Absence of major vessels.

2 ▶ Color—Arteries are brighter red than veins. They also have the arterial light reflex, a thin stripe of light down the middle.

3 ▶ A:V ratio—The ratio comparing the artery-to-vein width is 2:3 or 4:5.

Arteries too constricted.
Veins dilated.

4 ▶ A-V (arteriovenous) crossing— An artery and vein may cross paths. This is not significant if within 2 DD (Disc Diameters) of disc and if no sign of interruption in blood flow. There should be no indenting or displacing of vessel.

Crossings more than 2 DD away. Nicking or pinching of underlying vessel.
Vessel engorged peripheral to crossing.

5 ▶ Tortuosity—Mild vessel twisting when present in both eyes is usually congenital and not significant.

Extreme tortuosity or markedly asymmetric in two eyes.

NORMAL RANGE OF FINDINGS	ABNORMAL FINDINGS

7 ▶ Pulsations—Present in veins near the disc as their drainage meets the intermittent pressure of arterial systole. (Often hard to see.)

Absent pulsations.
(See Table 11–12, p. 359, in Jarvis: *Physical Examination and Health Assessment.*)

General Background of the Fundus. The color normally varies from light red to dark brown-red, generally corresponding with the person's skin color. There should be no lesions obstructing the retinal structures.

Abnormal lesions: hemorrhages, exudates, microaneurysms.

Macula. The macula is 1 DD in size and located 2 DD temporal to the disc. Inspect this area last in the funduscopic examination. A bright light on this area of central vision causes some watering, discomfort, and pupillary constriction. Note that the normal color of the area is somewhat darker than the rest of the fundus but even and homogeneous. Clumped pigment may occur with aging.

Clumped pigment occurs with trauma or retinal detachment.
    Hemorrhage or exudate in the macula occurs with senile macular degeneration.

DEVELOPMENTAL CONSIDERATIONS

Infants and Children

With a newborn, test *light perception* using the blink reflex; the neonate blinks in response to bright light. The pupillary light reflex also shows that the pupils constrict in response to light.

Absent blinking.
    Absent pupillary light reflex, especially after 3 weeks, indicates blindness.

Testing for strabismus (squint, crossed eye) is an important screening measure during early childhood. Untreated strabismus can lead to permanent visual damage, called *amblyopia ex anopsia.* Early recognition and treatment are essential. Diagnosis after age 6 years has a poor prognosis.

Check the *corneal light reflex* by shining a light toward the child's eyes. The light should be reflected at exactly the same spot in the two corneas. Some asymmetry (where one light falls off center) under age 6 months is normal.

Asymmetry in the corneal light reflex after 6 months is abnormal and must be referred.

NORMAL RANGE OF FINDINGS	ABNORMAL FINDINGS

Many infants have an *epicanthal fold,* an excess skin fold extending over the inner corner of the eye, partly or totally overlapping the inner canthus. This occurs frequently in Asian children and in 20 percent of whites. In non-Asians it disappears as the child grows, usually by age 10 years. While they are present, epicanthal folds give a false appearance of malalignment, called *pseudostrabismus,* yet the corneal light reflex is normal.

Asian infants normally have an upward slant of the palpebral fissures. Entropion, a turning inward of the eyelid, is normally found in some Asian children. If the lashes do not abrade the cornea, it is not significant.

Mongolian slant — An upward lateral slope together with epicanthal folds and hypertelorism (large spacing between the eyes) occurs with Down syndrome.

The Aging Adult

The eyebrows may show a loss of the outer one-third to one-half of hair. The remaining brow hair is coarse. Due to atrophy of elastic tissue, the skin around the eyes may show wrinkles or crow's feet. The upper lid may be so elongated as to rest on the lashes. (Table 7–1).

The eyes may appear sunken due to atrophy of the orbital fat. The orbital fat may also herniate, causing bulging at the lower lids and inner third of the upper lids.

Atrophy of the levator palpebrae muscle causes a partial ptosis. In contrast with the baggy lids previously described, ptosis is an actual drooping.

The lower lid may drop away from the globe, *ectropion.* This compromises the globe structures because the tears cannot drain into the out-turned puncta. Alternately, *entropion,* or a turning inward of the lower lid, may irritate the eye from friction of lashes.

Tear production may decrease, causing the eyes to look dry and lusterless with the person reporting a burning sensation. *Pingueculae*

See ectropion and entropion (see Table 7–2, pages 67–68).

NORMAL RANGE OF FINDINGS	ABNORMAL FINDINGS

commonly show on the sclera (see Table 7–1). These yellowish elevated nodules are due to a thickening of the bulbar conjunctiva from prolonged exposure to sun, wind, and dust. Pingueculae appear at the 3 and 9 o'clock positions, first on the nasal side, then on the temporal side.

The cornea may look cloudy with age. *Arcus senilis* is commonly seen around the cornea (see Table 7–1). This is a gray-white arc or circle around the limbus due to deposit of lipid material. As more lipid accumulates, the cornea may look thickened and raised, but the arcus has no affect on vision.

Xanthelasma are soft, raised, yellow plaques occurring on the lids of the inner canthus (see Table 7–1). These commonly occur around the fifth decade of life and more frequently in women. Xanthelasma occur with both high and normal blood levels of cholesterol and have no pathologic significance.

Pupils are small, and the pupillary light reflex may be slowed. The lens loses transparency and appears opaque.

In the ocular fundus, the blood vessels appear pale, narrow, and attenuated. Arterioles appear pale and straight, with a narrow light reflex. More arteriovenous (AV) crossing defects occur.

A normal development on the retinal surface are *drusen,* or benign degenerative hyaline deposits. They are small, round, yellow dots that are scattered haphazardly on the retina. Although they do not occur in a pattern, drusen are usually symmetrically placed in the two eyes. They have no affect on vision.

Drusen are easily confused with the abnormal finding of *hard exudates.* (See Table 11–13, p. 360, in Jarvis: *Physical Examination and Health Assessment.*)

Table 7–1 ► Aging Eye Changes

Relaxation of skin of upper eyelid

Pinguecula

Arcus senilis

Xanthelasma

ABNORMAL FINDINGS

Table 7-2 ▶ Abnormalities in the Eyelids

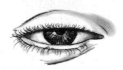

EXOPHTHALMOS (PROTRUDING EYES)

Exophthalmos is a forward displacement associated with thyroid disease. Note "lid lag," the upper lid rests well above the limbus and white sclera is visible.

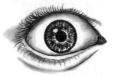

ECTROPION

The lower lid is loose and rolling out, does not approximate to eyeball. Puncta cannot siphon tears effectively so excess tearing results. Exposed palpebral conjunctiva increases risk for inflammation.

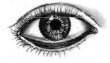

HORDEOLUM (STY)

Hordeolum is a localized staphylococcal infection of the hair follicles at the lid margin. It is painful, red, and swollen and resembles a pustule at the lid margin.

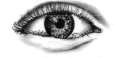

PTOSIS (DROOPING UPPER LID)

Ptosis occurs from neuromuscular weakness (e.g., myasthenia gravis), oculomotor cranial nerve III damage, or sympathetic nerve damage (e.g., Horner's syndrome).

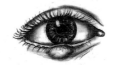

ENTROPION

The lower lid rolls in due to spasm of lids or contraction of scar tissue. Lashes may irritate cornea.

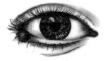

CHALAZION

A beady nodule protruding on the lid, chalazion is an infection or retention cyst of a meibomian gland. It is a nontender, firm, discrete swelling with freely moveable skin overlying the nodule. If it becomes inflamed, it points inside and not on the lid margin (in contrast with sty).

Table 7-2 ► Abnormalities in the Eyelids *Continued*

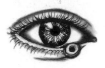

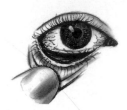

BASAL CELL CARCINOMA

Carcinoma is rare, but it occurs most often on the lower lid. It looks like a papule with an ulcerated center. Note the rolled out pearly edges.

CONJUNCTIVITIS

Infection of the conjunctiva shows red, beefy looking vessels at periphery but looks clearer around iris. This is a common disorder due to bacterial or viral infection, allergy, or chemical irritant. Purulent discharge accompanies bacterial infection. Often, the person has a history of an upper respiratory infection (URI).

Table 7-3 ► Abnormalities in the Pupil

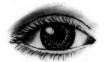

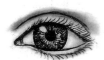

UNEQUAL PUPIL SIZE—ANISOCORIA

Although this exists normally in 5 percent of the population, consider central nervous system disease.

MONOCULAR BLINDNESS

When light is directed to the blind eye, there is no response. When light is directed to normal eye, both pupils constrict (direct and consensual response to light) as long as the oculomotor nerve is intact.

Table 7–3 ▶ Abnormalities in the Pupil *Continued*

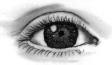

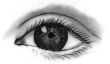

**CONSTRICTED AND FIXED PUPILS—
MIOSIS**

Miosis occurs with the use of pilocar-
pine drops for glaucoma treatment, the
use of narcotics, with iritis, and with
brain damage of pons.

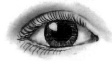

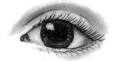

DILATED AND FIXED PUPILS—MYDRIASIS

Enlarged pupils occur with stimulation
of the sympathetic nervous system, reaction of sympathomimetic drugs, use
of dilating drops, acute glaucoma, past
or recent trauma. Enlarged pupils may
also indicated central nervous system
injury, circulatory arrest, or deep anesthesia.

☑ SUMMARY CHECKLIST

1 ▶ Test visual acuity
Snellen eye chart
Near vision (those older than
40 years or those having diffi-
culty reading)
2 ▶ Test visual fields—confronta-
tion test
3 ▶ Inspect extraocular muscle
(EOM) function
Corneal light reflex
Diagnostic positions test
4 ▶ Inspect external eye structures
General
Eyebrows
Eyelids and lashes
Eyeball alignment
Conjunctiva and sclera

5 ▶ Inspect anterior eyeball struc-
tures
Cornea and lens
Iris and pupil
Pupillary light reflex
Accommodation
6 ▶ Inspect the ocular fundus
Optic disc (color, shape, mar-
gins, cup-disc ratio)
Retinal vessels (number, color,
artery/vein (A/V) ratio, caliber,
arteriovenous crossings, tortu-
osity, pulsations)
General background (color, in-
tegrity)
Macula

Nursing Diagnoses Commonly Associated with the Eyes and Visual Disorders

Sensory/perceptual alteration: visual

Anxiety

Pain

Self-care deficit

Impaired home maintenance management

Diversional activity deficit

CHAPTER

8 Ears

The ear is the sensory organ for hearing and maintaining equilibrium. The external ear is the *auricle*, or *pinna*, and consists of movable cartilage and skin (Fig. 8–1).

The external ear funnels sound into its opening, the *external auditory canal* (Fig. 8–2). The canal is a cul-de-sac 2.5 to 3 cm long in the adult and has a slight S-curve.

The middle ear is a tiny air-filled cavity inside the temporal bone, and it contains the tiny auditory ossicles: the *malleus, incus,* and *stapes.*

The inner ear contains the *bony labyrinth*, which holds the sensory organs for equilibrium and hearing.

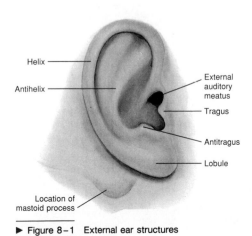

Helix

Antihelix

External auditory meatus

Tragus

Antitragus

Lobule

Location of mastoid process

▶ Figure 8–1　External ear structures

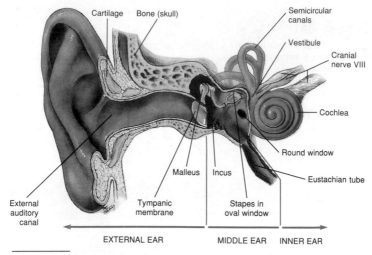

▶ Figure 8-2   Internal ear structures

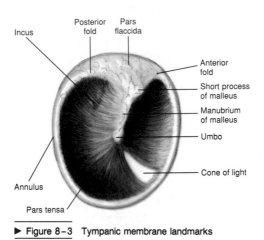

▶ Figure 8-3   Tympanic membrane landmarks

The *tympanic membrane* separates the external and middle ear (Fig. 8-3). It is translucent, with a pearly gray color and a prominent cone of light in the anteroinferior quadrant, which is the reflection of the otoscope light.

The parts of the malleus show through the translucent drum; these are the *umbo,* the *manubrium,* and the *short process.*

TRANSCULTURAL CONSIDERATIONS

 Cerumen is genetically determined and comes in two major types: (1) dry cerumen, which is gray, flaky, and frequently forms a thin mass in the ear canal, and (2) wet cerumen, which is honey to dark brown and moist. Asians and Native Americans have an 84 percent frequency of dry cerumen whereas blacks have a 99 percent and whites a 97 percent frequency of wet cerumen (Overfield, 1985).

Middle ear infection (otitis media) is one of the most common illnesses in children. The incidence and severity are increased in Native American and Alaskan and Canadian Eskimos. American black children have less incidence of otitis media than American white children (Bluestone and Klein, 1988).

SUBJECTIVE DATA

Earaches
Infections
Discharge
Hearing loss

Environmental noise
Tinnitus
Vertigo
Self-care behaviors
(hearing last checked,
method of cleaning ears)

OBJECTIVE DATA

Equipment Needed

Otoscope with bright light (fresh batteries give off white, not yellow, light)

Pneumatic bulb attachment, sometimes used with infant or young child

Tuning forks in 512, 1024 Hz

Preparation

Position the adult sitting up straight with his or her head at your eye level.

METHOD OF EXAMINATION

NORMAL RANGE OF FINDINGS	ABNORMAL FINDINGS
THE EXTERNAL EAR	
Inspect and Palpate the External Ear	
Size and Shape	
The ears are of equal size bilaterally with no swelling or thickening.	*Microtia*—ears smaller than 4 cm vertically

NORMAL RANGE OF FINDINGS	ABNORMAL FINDINGS
	Macrotia—ears larger than 10 cm vertically Edema

Skin Condition

The skin is intact, with no lumps or lesions. *Darwin's tubercle,* a small painless nodule at the helix, is sometimes present. This is a congenital variation and is not significant.	Reddened, excessively warm skin indicates inflammation. Crusts and scaling occur with otitis externa and with eczema, contact dermatitis, and seborrhea. Enlarged tender lymph nodes in the region indicate inflammation of the pinna or mastoid process. Tophi, sebaceous crust, chondrodermatitis, keloid, carcinoma. (See Table 12–2, pp. 388–389, in Jarvis: *Physical Examination and Health Assessment*).

Tenderness

The pinna and the tragus should feel firm and movement should produce no pain. Palpating the mastoid process should be painless.	Pain with movement occurs with otitis externa and furuncle. Pain at the mastoid process may indicate mastoiditis or lymphadenitis of the posterior auricular node.

The External Auditory Meatus

There should be no swelling, redness, or discharge.	Atresia—absence or closure of the ear canal. A sticky yellow discharge accompanies otitis externa, or it may indicate otitis media if the drum has ruptured. Impacted cerumen is a common cause of conductive hearing loss.
Some cerumen is usually present. The color varies from gray-yellow to light brown and black, and the texture varies from moist and waxy to dry and desiccated.	

NORMAL RANGE OF FINDINGS	ABNORMAL FINDINGS

THE OTOSCOPIC EXAMINATION

Inspect, Using the Otoscope

Choose the largest speculum that will fit comfortably. Tilt the person's head slightly away from you toward the opposite shoulder. This method brings the obliquely sloping eardrum into better view.

Pull the pinna up and back on an adult or older child; this helps straighten the S-shape of the canal. (Pull the pinna down on an infant and child under 3 years of age).

Hold the otoscope "upside down" along your fingers, and have the dorsa (back) of your hand along the person's cheek braced to steady the otoscope. (see Fig. 8-4 on p. 78).

The External Canal

Note any redness and swelling, lesions, foreign bodies, or discharge. If any discharge is present, note the color and odor. (Also clean any discharge off the speculum before examining the other ear to avoid contamination with possibly infectious material.) For a person with a hearing aid, note any irritation on the canal wall from poorly fitting earmolds.

Redness and swelling occur with otitis externa; canal may be completely closed with swelling.

Purulent otorrhea suggests otitis externa, or otitis media may be indicated if the drum has ruptured.

Frank blood or clear watery drainage (cerebrospinal fluid leak) following trauma suggests basal skull fracture and warrants immediate referral. Cerebrospinal fluid feels oily and produces a positive glucose finding on Tes-Tape.

Foreign body, exostosis, polyp, furuncle (see Table 12-3, pp. 389-391, in Jarvis: *Physical Examination and Health Assessment*).

The Tympanic Membrane

Color and Characteristics

The normal eardrum is shiny and translucent, with a pearl-gray color (see Fig. 8-3). The cone-shaped light reflex is prominent in the anterior

Yellow-amber color of the drum occurs with serous otitis media.

Red color occurs with acute otitis media.

NORMAL RANGE OF FINDINGS	ABNORMAL FINDINGS

inferior quadrant (at 5 o'clock in the right drum and 7 o'clock in the left drum). This is the reflection of the otoscope light. Sections of the malleus are visible through the translucent drum: the umbo, manubrium, and short process. (Infrequently, the incus behind the drum shows as a whitish haze in the upper posterior area). At the periphery, the annulus looks whiter and denser.

Absent or distorted landmarks.
Air/fluid level or air bubbles behind drum indicate serous otitis media (see Table 8–1 on p. 80).

Position

The eardrum is flat, slightly pulled in at the center, and flutters when the person performs the Valsalva maneuver or holds the nose and swallows (insufflation). These maneuvers assess drum mobility. Avoid them with an aging person because they may disrupt equilibrium. Also avoid middle ear insufflation in a person with upper respiratory infection because it could propel infectious matter into the middle ear.

Retracted drum due to vacuum in middle ear.
Bulging drum from increased pressure.
Drum does not move (see Table 8–1).

Integrity of Membrane

The normal tympanic membrane is intact. Some adults may show scarring, or a dense white patch on the drum, as sequela of repeated ear infections.

Perforation shows as a dark oval area or as a larger opening on the drum. (see Table 8–1).
Vesicles on drum.

HEARING ACUITY

Test Hearing Acuity

Voice Test

Test one ear at a time while masking hearing in the other ear by placing one finger on the tragus and rapidly pushing it in and out of the auditory meatus. Shield your lips. With your head 30 to 60 cm (1–2 ft) from the person's ear, exhale and whisper slowly some two-syllable words, such as Tuesday, armchair, baseball, and fourteen. Normally, the person repeats each word correctly after you say it.

The person is unable to hear whispered words. A whisper is a high-frequency sound and is used to detect high-tone loss.

NORMAL RANGE OF FINDINGS	ABNORMAL FINDINGS

Tuning Fork Tests

Tuning fork tests measure hearing by air conduction (AC) or bone conduction (BC) in which the sound vibrates through the cranial bones to the inner ear. The AC route through the ear canal and middle ear is usually the more sensitive route.

The *Weber test* is valuable when a person reports hearing better with one ear than the other. Place a vibrating turning fork in the midline of the person's skull and ask if the tone sounds the same in both ears or better in one. The person should hear the tone by bone conduction through the skull, and it should sound equally loud in both ears.

Sound lateralizes to one ear. (See Table 12–6, pp. 395–396, in Jarvis: *Physical Examination and Health Assessment*).

The *Rinne test* compares AC and BC sound. Place the stem of the vibrating tuning fork on the person's mastoid process and ask him or her to signal when the sound goes away. Quickly invert the fork so the vibrating end is near the ear canal; the person should still hear a sound. Normally, the sound is heard twice as long by AC (next to the ear canal) as by BC (through the mastoid process). A normal response is a positive Rinne test, or "AC > BC." Repeat with the other ear.

Ratio of AC to BC is altered with hearing loss.
Sound is heard longer by bone conduction.

DEVELOPMENTAL CONSIDERATIONS

Infants and Young Children

The top of the pinna should match an imaginary line extending from the corner of the eye to the occiput, and the ear should be positioned within 10 degrees of vertical.

Low-set ears or deviation in alignment may indicate mental retardation or a genitourinary malformation.

Remember to pull the pinna straight down on an infant or child under 3 years old. This method will match the slope of the ear canal.

When examining an infant or young child, a pneumatic bulb attachment enables you to direct a light puff of air toward the drum to assess vibratility (Fig. 8–4). For a

NORMAL RANGE OF FINDINGS	ABNORMAL FINDINGS

secure seal, choose the largest speculum that will fit the ear canal without causing pain. A rubber tip on the end of the speculum gives a better seal. Give a small pump to the bulb (positive pressure), then release the bulb (negative pressure). Normally, the tympanic membrane moves inward with a slight puff and outward with a slight release.

An abnormal response is no movement. Drum hypomobility indicates effusion or a high vacuum in the middle ear. For the newborn's first 6 weeks, drum immobility is the best indicator of middle ear infection.

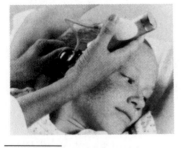

▶ Figure 8–4   Using otoscope with pneumatic bulb attachment

Normally, the tympanic membrane is intact. In a child being treated for chronic otitis media, you may note the presence of a myringotomy tube in the central part of the drum. This is inserted surgically to equalize pressure and drain secretions. Note a foreign body in a child's canal, such as a small stone or a bead.

Foreign body. (See Table 12–3, pp. 389–391, in Jarvis: *Physical Examination and Health Assessment*).

The Aging Adult

Earlobes may be pendulous with linear wrinkling. Coarse, wiry hairs may be present at the opening of the ear canal. During otoscopy, the drum may normally be whiter in color and more opaque, duller than in the younger adult: it also may look thickened. A high-tone frequency hearing loss is apparent for those affected with *presbycusis*,

NORMAL RANGE OF FINDINGS	ABNORMAL FINDINGS

hearing loss that occurs with aging. This condition is revealed by difficulty hearing whispered words in the voice test and difficulty hearing consonants during conversational speech.

For more information on assessment of the ears and hearing, see Chapter 12 in Jarvis: *Physical Examination and Health Assessment,* pp. 364–397.

A B N O R M A L   F I N D I N G S

Table 8-1 ► Abnormalities of the Tympanic Membrane

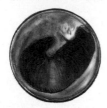

RETRACTED DRUM

Landmarks look more prominent. Malleus handle looks shorter and more horizontal. Short process very prominent. Light reflex absent or distorted. Drum is dull and lusterless and does not move. Signs indicate obstructed eustachian tube and serous otitis media.

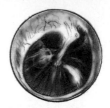

SEROUS OTITIS MEDIA

An amber-yellow drum, an air/fluid level with fine black dividing line, or air bubbles visible behind drum. Symptoms are feeling of fullness, transient hearing loss, popping sound with swallowing. Also called: Secretory otitis media, middle ear effusion, glue ear.

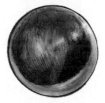

ACUTE PURULENT OTITIS MEDIA

An absent light reflex is an early sign. Redness and bulging are first noted in superior part of drum (pars flaccida), along with earache and fever. Then fiery red bulging of entire drum occurs; deep throbbing pain; fever; transient hearing loss. Pneumatic otoscopy reveals drum hypomobility.

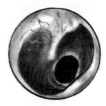

PERFORATION

Drum rupture from increased pressure or from trauma. Appears as a round or oval darkened area on the drum. *Central* perforations occur in the pars tensa, *marginal* perforations at the annulus.

☑ SUMMARY CHECKLIST

1 ▶ Inspect external ear
  A. Size and shape of auricle
  B. Position and alignment on head
  C. Note skin condition—color, lumps, lesions
  D. Check movement of auricle and tragus for tenderness
  E. Evaluate external auditory meatus. Note size, swelling, redness, discharge, cerumen, lesions, foreign bodies
2 ▶ Otoscopic examination
  A. External canal
    1. Cerumen, discharge, foreign bodies, lesions
    2. Redness or swelling of canal wall
  B. Inspect tympanic membrane
    1. Color and characteristics
    2. Note position (flat, bulging, retracted)
    3. Integrity of membrane
3 ▶ Test hearing acuity
  A. Note behavioral response to conversational speech
  B. Voice test
  C. Tuning fork tests—Weber and Rinne

Nursing Diagnoses Commonly Associated with the Ears and Hearing Disorders

Sensory/perceptual alteration: auditory

Impaired verbal communication

Pain

CHAPTER

9 Nose, Mouth, and Throat

ANATOMY

The nose is the first segment of the respiratory system. It warms, moistens, and filters the inhaled air, and it is the sensory organ for smell.

The oval openings at the base of the nose are the *nares* (Fig. 9–1). The *columella* divides the two nares and is continuous inside with the nasal septum.

Inside, the nasal cavity is large and extends back over the roof of the mouth (Fig. 9–2). Nasal mucosa appears redder than oral mucosa because of the rich blood supply present to warm the inhaled air.

The lateral walls of each nasal cavity contain three bony projections—the *turbinates*. They increase the surface area so that more blood vessels are available to warm, humidify and filter the inhaled air.

The mouth is the first segment of the digestive system and an airway for the respiratory system (Fig. 9-3). It contains the teeth and gums, tongue, and three pairs of salivary glands.

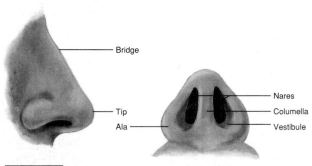

▶ Figure 9–1   External nose structures

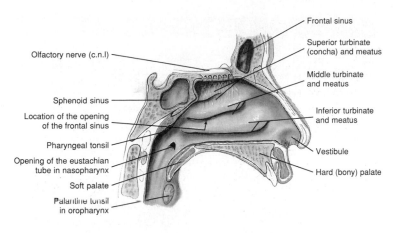

LEFT LATERAL WALL — NASAL CAVITY

▶ Figure 9–2 Internal nose structures

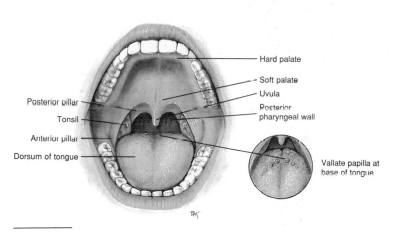

▶ Figure 9–3 Mouth structures

TRANSCULTURAL CONSIDERATIONS

Bifid uvula, a condition in which the uvula is split either completely or partially, is common in Native American groups and Asians and is rare in whites and blacks.

Cleft lip and *cleft palate* are most common in Asians and Native Americans and least common in blacks. *Torus palatinus,* a bony ridge running the middle of the hard palate, is very common in Native Americans and in Eskimos and Asians.

S U B J E C T I V E   D A T A

Nose

Discharge

Frequent colds (upper respiratory infections)

Sinus pain

Trauma

Epistaxis

Allergies

Altered smell

Mouth and Throat

Sores or lesions

Sore throat

Bleeding gums

Toothache

Hoarseness

Dysphagia

Altered taste

Self-care behaviors

    Dental care pattern

    Dentures or appliances

O B J E C T I V E   D A T A

Equipment Needed

Otoscope with short, wide-tipped nasal speculum attachment or nasal speculum and penlight

Tongue blade

Cotton gauze pad (4 × 4 inches)

Gloves

Preparation

Position the person sitting up straight with his or her head at your eye level. Remove dentures.

METHOD OF EXAMINATION

NORMAL RANGE OF FINDINGS	ABNORMAL FINDINGS

THE NOSE

Inspect and Palpate the Nose

The nose is symmetric, in the midline, and in proportion to other facial features. Inspect for any deformity, asymmetry, inflammation, or skin lesions.

NORMAL RANGE OF FINDINGS	ABNORMAL FINDINGS

Test the patency of the nostrils. This reveals any obstruction which later is explored using the nasal speculum.

Absence of sniff indicates obstruction.

Nasal Cavity

Attach the short, wide-tipped speculum to the otoscope head and insert into the nasal vestibule, avoiding pressure on the nasal septum.

Inspect the nasal mucosa, noting its normal red color and smooth moist surface (Fig. 9–4). Note any swelling, discharge, bleeding, or foreign body.

Rhinitis—nasal mucosa is swollen and bright red with an upper respiratory infection.

Discharge is common with rhinitis and sinusitis, varying from watery and copious to thick, purulent, and green-yellow.

With chronic allergy, mucosa looks swollen, boggy, pale, and gray.

For more information and illustrations on abnormalities of the nose see Table 13-1, pp. 430–432 in Jarvis: *Physical Examination and Health Assessment.* A deviated septum looks like a hump or shelf in one nasal cavity.

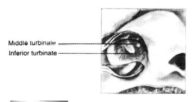

Middle turbinate
Inferior turbinate

▶ Figure 9–4   Viewing the naris through nasal speculum

Observe the nasal septum for deviation, perforation, or bleeding. A deviated septum is common and not significant unless air flow is obstructed.

Perforation is seen as a spot of light from penlight shining in other naris.

Epistaxis commonly comes from anterior septum.

Inspect the turbinates, the bony ridges curving down from the lateral walls. The middle and inferior turbinates appear the same light red color as the nasal mucosa. Note any swelling but do not try to push the speculum past it. Turbinates are quite vascular and tender if touched.

Note any polyps, benign growths that accompany chronic allergy, and distinguish them from normal turbinates.

Polyps are smooth, pale gray in color, avascular, mobile, and nontender.

THE SINUS AREAS

Palpate the Sinus Areas

Using your thumbs, press over the frontal sinuses below the eyebrows

NORMAL RANGE OF FINDINGS	ABNORMAL FINDINGS

and over the maxillary sinuses below the cheekbones. Do not press directly on the eyeballs. The person should feel firm pressure but no pain.

Sinus areas are tender to palpation in persons with chronic allergies and acute infection (sinusitis).

THE MOUTH
Inspect the Mouth

Lips

Inspect the lips for color, moisture, cracking, or lesions. Black persons may have bluish lips which is normal.

In light-skinned people: circumoral pallor occurs with shock and anemia, cyanosis with hypoxemia and chilling, cherry red lips with carbon monoxide poisoning, acidosis from aspirin poisoning, or ketoacidosis.

Cheilosis, cracking at the corners.

Herpes simplex, other lesions (see Table 9–1 on pp. 90–91).

Teeth and Gums

Teeth normally appear white, straight, evenly spaced, and clean and free of debris or decay. Note any diseased, absent, loose, or abnormally positioned teeth.

Ask the person to bite and note alignment of upper and lower jaw. Normal occlusion in the back is the upper teeth resting directly on the lowers; in the front, the upper incisors slightly override the lower incisors.

Normally, the gums look pink or coral with a stippled (dotted) surface. The gum margins are tight and well defined. Check for swelling, retraction of gingival margins, and spongy, bleeding, or discolored gums. Black people may normally have a dark, melanotic line along the gingival margin.

Discolored teeth: appear brown with excessive fluoride use, yellow with tobacco use.

Grinding down of tooth surface.

Plaque—soft debris.

Caries—decay.

Malocclusion, e.g., protrusion of upper or lower incisors.

Gingival hypertrophy, crevices between teeth and gums, pockets of debris.

Gums bleed with slight pressure.

Dark line on gingival margins occurs with lead and bismuth poisoning.

Tongue

The tongue color is pink and even. The dorsal surface is normally roughened from the papillae. A thin, white coating may be present. Ask the person to touch the tongue to

Beefy red swollen tongue. Smooth glossy areas (see Table 13–5, pp. 346–348 in Jarvis: *Physical Examination and Health Assessment*).

NORMAL RANGE OF FINDINGS	ABNORMAL FINDINGS
the roof of the mouth. Its ventral surface looks smooth, glistening, and shows veins. Saliva is present.	Enlarged tongue occurs with mental retardation, hypothyroidism, acromegaly. Dry mouth occurs with dehydration, fever; tongue has deep vertical fissures. Excessive saliva and drooling.
Carefully inspect the entire U-shaped area under the tongue and the tongue. Note any white patches, nodules, or ulcerations. If lesions are present or with any person over 50 or with a positive history of smoking or alcohol use, put on a glove and palpate the area. Notice any induration.	Any lesion or ulcer persisting for more than 2 weeks must be investigated. An indurated area may be a mass or lymphadenopathy and must be investigated.

Buccal Mucosa

The buccal mucosa looks pink, smooth, and moist although patchy hyperpigmentation is common and normal in dark-skinned people.	Dappled brown patches present with Addison's disease (chronic adrenal insufficiency).
Stensen's duct, the opening of the parotid salivary gland, looks like a small dimple opposite the upper second molar. You may also see a raised occlusion line on the buccal mucosa parallel with the level the teeth meet: this is due to the teeth closing against the cheek.	Orifice of Stensen's duct looks red with mumps. Koplik's spots—a prodromal sign of measles.
Fordyce's granules are small, isolated white or yellow papules on the mucosa of the cheek, tongue, and lips. These little sebaceous cysts are painless and not significant.	The chalky white raised patch of *leukoplakia* is abnormal. (See Table 13–4, pp. 435–436 in Jarvis: *Physical Examination and Health Assessment*).

Palate

The more anterior hard palate is white with irregular transverse rugae. The posterior soft palate is pink, smooth, and upwardly movable. A common variation is a nodular bony ridge down the middle of the hard palate, a *torus palatinus* (see Table 9–1).	The hard palate appears yellow with jaundice. In blacks with jaundice, it may look yellow, muddy yellow, or green-brown.
Ask the person to say "ahhh" and note the soft palate and uvula rise in the midline. This tests one function of cranial nerve X, the vagus nerve.	A *bifid* uvula appears as if split in two; more common in Native Americans (see Table 13–6, p. 438 in Jarvis: *Physical Examination and Health Assessment*).

NORMAL RANGE OF FINDINGS	ABNORMAL FINDINGS

THE THROAT
Inspect the Throat

The *tonsils* are the same pink as the oral mucosa, and their surface is peppered with indentations or crypts. There should be no exudate on the tonsils. Tonsils are graded in size as:
1+—visible;
2+—halfway between tonsillar pillars and uvula;
3+—touching the uvula;
4+—touching each other
　You may normally see 1+ or 2+ tonsils in healthy people, especially in children.
　Depress the tongue with a tongue blade. Scan the posterior pharyngeal wall for color, exudate, or lesions. When finished, discard the tongue blade.
　Touching the posterior wall with the tongue blade elicits the gag reflex. This tests cranial nerves IX and X. Test cranial nerve XII, the hypoglossal nerve, by asking the person to stick out the tongue. It should protrude in the midline. Children enjoy this request. Note any tremor, loss of movement, or deviation to the side.
　Notice any breath odor, *halitosis.* This is common and usually due to a local cause, such as poor oral hygiene, consumption of odoriferous foods, alcohol consumption, heavy smoking, or dental infection. Occasionally, it may indicate a systemic disease.

With an acute infection, tonsils are bright red, swollen, and may have exudate or large white spots. A white membrane covering the tonsils may accompany infectious mononucleosis, leukemia and diphtheria.

Tonsils are enlarged to 2+, 3+, or 4+, with an acute infection.

With damage to cranial nerve XII, the tongue deviates *toward* the paralyzed side.
　A fine tremor of the tongue occurs with hyperthyroidism, a coarse tremor with cerebral palsy and alcoholism.
Diabetic ketoacidosis has a sweet fruity breath odor; this acetone smell also occurs in children with malnutrition or dehydration. Others are an ammonia breath odor with uremia, a musty odor with liver disease, a foul, fetid odor with dental or respiratory infections, and alcohol odor with alcohol ingestion or chemicals.

DEVELOPMENTAL CONSIDERATIONS

Infants and Children

The newborn may have milia across the nose. The nasal bridge may be

Nasal flaring in the infant indicates respiratory distress.

NORMAL RANGE OF FINDINGS	ABNORMAL FINDINGS
flat in black and Asian children. There should be no nasal flaring or narrowing with breathing.	In a child with chronic allergy, a transverse ridge is present across the nose from wiping the nose upward with the palm. Nasal narrowing on inhalation is seen with chronic nasal obstruction and mouth-breathing.
Note the number of teeth, and whether or not it is appropriate for the child's age. Also note patterns of eruption, position, condition, and hygiene. Use this guide for children under 2 years; the child's age in months minus the number 6 should equal the expected number of deciduous teeth. Normally, all 20 deciduous teeth are in by 2½ years.	No teeth by age 1 year. Discolored teeth: appear yellow or yellow-brown with infants taking tetracycline or whose mothers took the drug during the last trimester; appear green or black with excessive iron ingestion, although this reverses when the iron is stopped. Malocclusion: upper or lower dental arches are out of alignment.
Note any bruising or laceration on the buccal mucosa or gums of infant or young child.	Trauma may indicate child abuse due to forced feeding of bottle or spoon.

The Pregnant Female

Gum hypertrophy (surface looks smooth and stippling disappears) may occur normally at puberty or during pregnancy (pregnancy gingivitis).

The Aging Adult

In the edentulous person, the mouth and lips fold in, giving a "purse-string" appearance. The teeth may look slightly yellowed though the color is uniform. The teeth may look longer as the gum margins recede.

Tooth surfaces look worn down or abraded. Old dental work deteriorates, especially at the gum margins. The teeth loosen with bone resorption and may move with palpation.

The tongue looks smoother due to papillary atrophy. The aging adult's buccal mucosa is thinned and may look shinier as though it were "varnished."

ABNORMAL FINDINGS

Table 9–1 ▶ Abnormalities of the Mouth and Throat

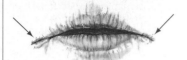

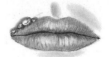

CHEILOSIS (ANGULAR STOMATITIS, PERLECHE)

Painful fissures at the corners of the mouth occur with excess salivation and monilial infection. Seen in edentulous persons and those with poorly fitting dentures that cause folding in of corners of mouth.

HERPES SIMPLEX I

Cold sores are groups of clear vesicles with a surrounding erythematous base. These evolve into pustules or crusts and heal in 4 to 10 days. The most likely site is the lip-skin junction; infection often recurs in same site. It may be precipitated by sunlight, fever, colds, allergy.

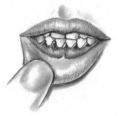

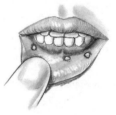

GINGIVITIS

Gum margins are red, swollen, and bleed easily. Note bulbous gingivae between the teeth. Inflammation is usually due to poor dental hygiene or vitamin C deficiency. The condition may occur in pregnancy and puberty due to change in hormonal balance.

APHTHOUS ULCERS

A "canker sore" appears first as a vesicle, then as a small, round ulcer with a white base surrounded by a red halo. It is quite painful and lasts for 1 to 2 weeks. The cause is unknown, although it is associated with stress, fatigue, and food allergy.

Table 9-1 ▶ Abnormalities of the Mouth and Throat *Continued*	
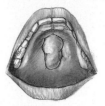	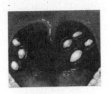
TORUS PALATINUS	**ACUTE TONSILLITIS AND PHARYNGITIS**
A normal variation is a nodular bony ridge down the middle of the hard palate. This benign growth arises after puberty and is more common in Native Americans, Eskimos, and Asians.	Bright red throat, swollen tonsils, white or yellow exudate on tonsils and pharynx, swollen uvula, and enlarged, tender cervical and tonsillar nodes. Accompanied by severe sore throat, high fever of sudden onset. (Caution: Cannot discriminate bacterial from viral infection on clinical data alone; need a throat culture).

☑ SUMMARY CHECKLIST

NOSE

1 ▶ Inspect external nose for symmetry, any deformity, or lesions.
2 ▶ Palpation—Test patency of each nostril.
3 ▶ Inspect using nasal speculum.
   A. Color and integrity of nasal mucosa.
   B. Septum—note any deviation, perforation, or bleeding.
   C. Turbinates—note color, any exudate, swelling, or polyps.
4 ▶ Palpate the sinus areas—note any tenderness.

MOUTH AND THROAT

1 ▶ Inspect using penlight.
   A. Lips, teeth, and gums, tongue, buccal mucosa. Note color, if structures are intact, any lesions.
   B. Palate and uvula—note integrity and mobility as person phonates.
   C. Grade tonsils.
   D. Pharyngeal wall—note color, any exudate, or lesions.
2 ▶ Palpation
   When indicated, palpation of mouth.

Nursing Diagnoses Commonly Associated with Nose, Mouth, Throat Disorders

Altered oral mucous membrane

Pain

Impaired swallowing

Ineffective airway clearance

Sensory/perceptual alteration:

  olfactory

  gustatory

10 Breasts and Axillae

ANATOMY

The female breasts are accessory reproductive organs whose function is to produce milk. The breasts lie anterior to the pectoralis major and serratus anterior muscles, between the second and sixth ribs (Fig. 10–1). The superior lateral corner of breast tissue, called the axillary *tail of Spence*, projects up and laterally into the axilla.

Internally, the breast is composed of (1) *glandular tissue*, containing 15 to 20 lobes radiating from the nipple (Fig. 10–2). Each lobe empties into a lactiferous duct and these converge toward the nipple. (2) The

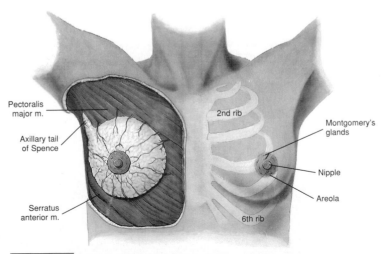

Pectoralis major m.

Axillary tail of Spence

Serratus anterior m.

2nd rib

Montgomery's glands

Nipple

Areola

6th rib

▶ Figure 10–1   Surface anatomy of the breast

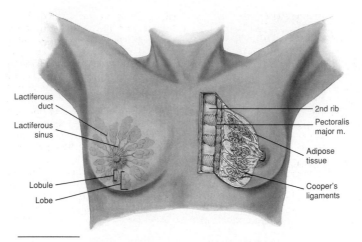

▶ Figure 10-2 Internal anatomy: (1) glandular tissue, (2) fibrous tissue including suspensory ligaments, (3) adipose tissue

spensory ligaments, or *Cooper's ligaments,* are fibrous bands extending vertically from the surface to the chest wall muscles. They support the breast. (3) The adipose, or fatty, tissue provides most of the bulk of the breast.

The breast has extensive lymphatic drainage (Fig. 10-3): (1) *central axillary* nodes, high up in the middle of the axilla; (2) *pectoral,* along the lateral edge of the pectoralis major muscle; (3) *subscapular,* along the lateral edge of the scapula; (4) *lateral,* along the humerus, inside the upper arm. From the central axillary nodes, drainage flows up to the infraclavicular and supraclavicular nodes.

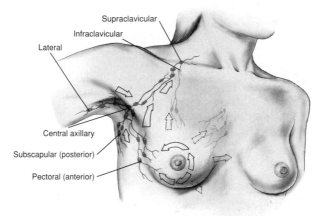

Arrows indicate direction of lymph flow

Figure 10-3 Lymphatic drainage

TRANSCULTURAL CONSIDERATIONS

 Racial differences in sexual maturity demonstrate that black girls develop secondary sex characteristics earlier than white girls of the same age (Harlan, 1980). Also, axillary hair appears earlier in black females, and Asian women normally have fine, sparse pubic hair.

The incidence of breast cancer varies with different cultural groups and may be related to a diet rich in fat. The high incidence of breast cancer rates in the United States, Britain, and the Netherlands correlates with a high amount of fat in the diet of those nations. In Japan, Peru, Singapore, and Romania, where people eat a lean diet, the incidence of breast cancer is one-sixth to one-half that of the United States (American Cancer Society, 1991). Migratory studies show, however, that when Japanese move to the United States, the previously low incidence of breast cancer rises as they adapt to a western diet (Secretary's Task Force on Black and Minority Health, 1986)

SUBJECTIVE DATA

Breast
Pain
Lump
Discharge
Rash
Swelling
Trauma
History of breast disease

Surgery
Perform breast self-exam
Last mammogram

Axilla
Tenderness
Lump or swelling
Rash

OBJECTIVE DATA

Equipment Needed
Small pillow
Ruler marked in centimeters
Pamphlet or teaching aid for breast self-examination

Preparation
The woman is sitting up, facing the examiner. Use a short gown, open at the back, and lift it up to the woman's shoulders during inspection. During palpation the woman is supine: cover one breast with the gown while examining the other.

METHOD OF EXAMINATION

NORMAL RANGE OF FINDINGS	ABNORMAL FINDINGS

THE BREASTS

Inspect the Breasts

General Appearance

Note symmetry of size and shape (common to have a slight asymmetry in size).

A sudden increase in size of one breast signifies inflammation or neoplasm.

Skin

The skin is normally smooth and of even color with no redness, bulging, dimpling, skin lesions, or focal vascular pattern. A fine blue vascular network is normally visible in lightly pigmented females during pregnancy. Pale linear striae, or stretch marks, often follow pregnancy.

Normally there is no edema. Edema exaggerates the hair follicles, giving a "pig skin" or "orange peel" look (also called *peau d'orange*).

Hyperpigmentation
Redness and heat with inflammation.
Unilateral dilated superficial veins in a nonpregnant woman.

Lymphatic Drainage Areas

The axillary and supraclavicular regions have no bulging, discoloration, or edema.

Nipple

The nipples should be symmetrically located and usually protrude, although some are flat and some inverted. Distinguish a recently retracted nipple from one that has been inverted for many years or since puberty.

Note any dry scaling, any fissure or ulceration, and bleeding or other discharge. Normally, there are none.

A normal variation in about 1 percent of men and women is *supernumerary nipple*, a congenital finding. Usually, it is 5 to 6 cm below the breast near the midline and looks like a mole, although a close look reveals a tiny nipple and areola. It is not significant.

Deviation in pointing.
Recent nipple retraction signifies acquired disease (see Table 14-3, pp. 468-469 in Jarvis: *Physical Examination and Health Assessment*).

Any discharge must be explored, especially in the presence of a breast mass.

Rarely, glandular tissue, a supernumerary breast, or polymastia, is present.

NORMAL RANGE OF FINDINGS	ABNORMAL FINDINGS

Maneuvers to Screen for Retraction

First ask the woman to lift arms slowly over the head. Both breasts should move up symmetrically.

Next ask her to put her hands onto her hips and then to push her two palms together. There will be a slight lifting of both breasts.

Retraction signs are due to fibrosis in the breast tissue, usually caused by growing neoplasms.
Note a lag in movement of one breast.
Note a dimpling or a pucker which indicates skin retraction (see Table 14–3, pp. 468–469 in Jarvis: *Physical Examination and Health Assessment*)

THE AXILLAE

Inspect and Palpate the Axillae

Inspect the skin, noting any rash or infection. Lift the woman's arm and support it yourself so that her muscles are loose and relaxed. Reach your fingers high into the axillae and move them firmly down in each direction.

Usually nodes are not palpable, although you may feel a small, soft, nontender node in the central group. Expect some tenderness when palpating high in the axillae. Note any enlarged and tender lymph nodes.

Nodes enlarge with any local infection of the breast, arm, or hand, and with breast cancer metastases.

BREAST PALPATION

Palpate the Breasts

Help the woman to a supine position. Tuck a small pad under the side to be palpated and raise her arm over her head to flatten the breast tissue and displace it medially.

Use the pads of your first three fingers and make a gentle rotary motion on the breast. Choose one of two patterns for palpation: (1) spokes-on-a-wheel (Fig. 10–4); (2) or, concentric circles, (Fig. 10–5). Take care to palpate the tail of Spence extending from the upper quadrant into the axillae.

NORMAL RANGE OF FINDINGS   ABNORMAL FINDINGS

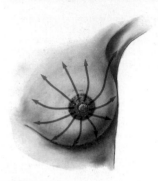

▶ Figure 10–4   Spokes-on-a-wheel pattern of palpation

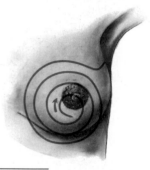

▶ Figure 10–5   Concentric circles pattern of palpation

In nulliparous women, normal breast tissue feels firm, smooth, and elastic. After pregnancy, the tissue feels softer and looser. Premenstrual engorgement is normal due to increasing progesterone and consists of a slight enlargement, a tenderness to palpation, and a generalized nodularity; the lobes feel prominent and their margins more distinct.

A firm transverse ridge of compressed tissue in the lower quadrants, the *inframammary ridge*, is especially noticeable in large breasts. Do not confuse it with an abnormal lump.

Heat, redness and swelling in nonlactating and nonpostpartum breasts indicate inflammation.

NORMAL RANGE OF FINDINGS	ABNORMAL FINDINGS

Palpate the nipple. Note any induration or subareolar mass. Use your thumb and forefinger to apply gentle pressure or a stripping action to the nipple. If any discharge appears, note its color and consistency.

If you feel a lump or mass, note these characteristics:

1. Location—diagram the breast in the woman's record and mark the location of the lump.
2. Size—in centimeters: width × length × thickness.
3. Shape—oval, round, lobulated, or indistinct.
4. Consistency—soft, firm or hard.
5. Movable—freely moveable or fixed.
6. Distinctness—solitary or multiple.
7. Nipple—displaced or retracted.
8. Skin over the lump—erythematous, dimpled, or retracted.
9. Tenderness—to palpation.
10. Lymphadenopathy.

Abnormal findings: Except in pregnancy and lactation, discharge is abnormal (see Table 14–6, pp. 471–472 in Jarvis: *Physical Examination and Health Assessment*).

See Tables 14–4 and 14–5, pp. 470–471 in Jarvis: *Physical Examination and Health Assessment,* for description of common breast lumps using these characteristics.

THE BREAST SELF-EXAMINATION

Help each woman establish a regular schedule of self-care. The best time to conduct breast self-examination is right after the menstrual period or the fourth day through seventh day of the menstrual cycle when the breasts are the smallest and least congested. Advise the pregnant or menopausal woman who is not having menstrual periods to select a familiar date to examine her breasts each month: for example, her birthdate or the day the rent is due.

Describe the correct technique, rationale, and expected findings. Teach the woman to do this in front of a mirror while she is disrobed to the waist. At home, she can start palpation in the shower where soap and water assist palpation. Palpation should then be performed while lying supine. Encourage the woman

NORMAL RANGE OF FINDINGS	ABNORMAL FINDINGS

to palpate her own breasts while you are there to monitor her technique. Use the return demonstration to assess her technique and understanding of the procedure.

THE MALE BREAST

Inspect the chest wall, noting the skin surface and any lumps or swelling. Palpate the nipple area for any lumps or tissue enlargement. It should feel even with no nodules.

The normal male breast has a flat disc of undeveloped breast tissue beneath the nipple. *Gynecomastia* is an enlargement of this breast tissue, making it clinically distinguishable from the other tissue in the chest wall. It feels like a smooth, firm, moveable disc. This occurs normally during puberty. It usually affects only one breast and is temporary.

Gynecomastia also occurs with some medications and some disease states (see Table 14–8, p. 473 in Jarvis: *Physical Examination and Health Assessment*).

DEVELOPMENTAL CONSIDERATIONS

Infants and Children

In the neonate, the breasts may be enlarged and may secrete a clear or white fluid called "witch's milk." These signs are not significant and are resolved within a few days to a few weeks.

The Adolescent

Adolescent breast development usually begins between 10 and 13 years of age. Expect some asymmetry during growth. Record the stage of development using Tanner's sex maturity ratings described in Table 10–1 on p. 102. Use the chart to teach normal developmental stages to the adolescent and assure her of her own normal progress.

With maturing adolescents, palpate the breasts as you would with the adult. The breasts normally feel firm and uniform. Note any mass.

Note precocious development occurring before age 8. It is usually normal but also occurs with thyroid dysfunction, stilbestrol ingestion, or ovarian or adrenal tumor.

Note delayed development occurring with hormonal failure, anorexia nervosa beginning before puberty, or severe malnutrition.

At this age, if a mass occurs, it is almost always a benign fibroadenoma, or a cyst.

NORMAL RANGE OF FINDINGS	ABNORMAL FINDINGS

The Pregnant Female

A delicate, blue vascular pattern is visible over the breasts of lightly pigmented females. The breasts increase in size as do the nipples. Jagged linear stretch marks, or striae, may develop if the breasts have a marked increase in size. The nipples also become darker and more erect. The areolae widen, grow darker, and contain small, scattered, elevated Montgomery's glands. On palpation, the breasts feel more nodular, and thick yellow colostrum can be expressed after the first trimester.

The Lactating Female

Colostrum changes to milk production around the third postpartum day. At this time, the breasts may become engorged, appear enlarged, reddened, and shiny, and feel warm and hard. Frequent nursing helps drain the ducts and sinuses and stimulates milk production.

Nipple soreness is normal, appears around the twentieth nursing day, lasts 24 to 48 hours, then disappears rapidly. The nipples may look red, irritated, and may even crack, but will heal rapidly if kept dry and exposed to air. Again, frequent nursing is the best treatment for nipple soreness.

One section of the breast surface appearing red and tender indicates a plugged duct (see Table 14–7, p. 472, in Jarvis: *Physical Examination and Health Assessment*).

The Aging Female

The breasts look pendulous, flattened, and sagging. Nipples may be retracted but can be pulled outward. The breasts feel more granular, and the terminal ducts around the nipple feel more prominent and stringy. Thickening of the inframammary ridge at the lower breast is normal and feels more prominent with age.

Reinforce the value of breast self-examination. Women over 50 years have an increased risk of breast cancer (Table 10–2).

Since atrophy causes shrinkage of normal glandular tissue, cancer detection is somewhat easier. Any palpable lump that cannot be positively identified as a normal structure should be referred.

Table 10-1 ► Sexual Maturity Rating in Girls

Stage

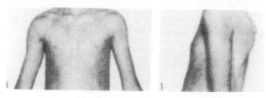

1 Preadolescent. Only a small elevated nipple.

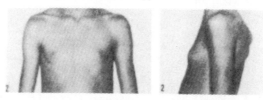

2 Breast bud stage. A small mound of breast and nipple develops. The areola widens.

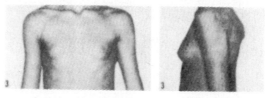

3 The breast and areola enlarge. The nipple is flush with the breast surface.

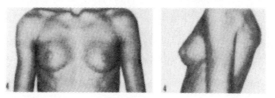

4 The areola and nipple form a secondary mound over the breast.

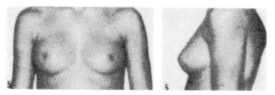

5 Mature breast; only the nipple protrudes, the areola is flush with the breast contour. (The areola may continue as a secondary mound in some normal women.)

Average breast development begins between 10 and 11 years of age (normal range between 8 and 13 years). The five stages of breast development follow the pattern described by Tanner's sexual maturity rating or SMR (Tanner, J.M.: Growth at Adolescence. Oxford, England: Blackwell Scientific, 1962).

Table 10-2 ► Breast Cancer Risk Factors

Documented hereditary cancer syndrome
Family history of breast cancer in first-degree relatives
Nulliparity or first childbirth after age 30
Early menarche and late menopause
Proliferative breast lesion (especially with atypical cells)
High-dose radiation exposure to the chest area
Hormone replacement therapy (in women at increased risk)*
High fat diet
Obesity (especially postmenopause)

   * Documented with total accumulated doses of more than 1,500 mg.
   (Reprinted by permission of the American Association of occupational Health
Nurses, AAOHN Journal, Vol. 37, No. 5.)

☑ SUMMARY CHECKLIST

1 ► Inspect breasts as the woman sits, raises arms over head, pushes hands on hips, leans forward.

2 ► Inspect the supraclavicular and infraclavicular areas.

3 ► Palpate the axillae and regional lymph nodes.

4 ► With woman supine, palpate the breast tissue including tail of Spence, the nipples, and areolae.

5 ► Teach breast self-examination.

Nursing Diagnoses Commonly Associated with Breast Disorders

Knowledge deficit: breast self-examination

Anxiety

Anticipatory grieving

Body image disturbance

Ineffective individual coping

Ineffective breastfeeding

Pain

11 Thorax and Lungs

ANATOMY

The thoracic cage is a bony structure with a conical shape (Fig. 11–1). It is defined by the sternum, 12 pairs of ribs, 12 thoracic vertebrae, and the diaphragm.

The *costochondral junctions* are the points at which the ribs join their cartilages. They are not palpable.

The *suprasternal notch* is the hollow U-shaped depression just above the sternum, in between the clavicles.

The *manubriosternal angle,* or "angle of Louis," is the articulation of the manubrium and body of the sternum, and it is continuous with the second rib. Each intercostal space is numbered by the rib above it.

The *costal angle* is formed by the right and left costal margins where they meet at the xiphoid process. It is usually 90 degrees or less.

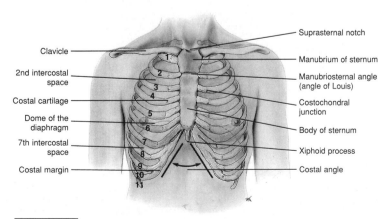

Clavicle

2nd intercostal space

Costal cartilage

Dome of the diaphragm

7th intercostal space

Costal margin

Suprasternal notch

Manubrium of sternum

Manubriosternal angle (angle of Louis)

Costochondral junction

Body of sternum

Xiphoid process

Costal angle

▶ Figure 11–1   Surface landmarks

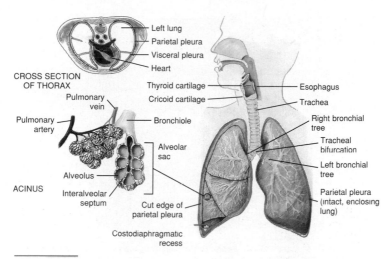

CROSS SECTION
OF THORAX

Left lung
Parietal pleura
Visceral pleura
Heart

Thyroid cartilage
Cricoid cartilage

Esophagus
Trachea

Pulmonary
vein

Pulmonary
artery

Bronchiole

Right bronchial
tree

Tracheal
bifurcation

Left bronchial
tree

Alveolar
sac

ACINUS

Alveolus

Interalveolar
septum

Cut edge of
parietal pleura

Parietal pleura
(intact, enclosing
lung)

Costodiaphragmatic
recess

▶ Figure 11–2   Trachea and bronchial tree

The trachea lies anterior to the esophagus and is 10 to 11 cm long in the adult (Fig. 11–2). It begins at the level of the cricoid cartilage in the neck and bifurcates just below the sternal angle into the right and left main bronchi.

An *acinus* is a functional respiratory unit and consists of the bronchioles and alveoli. Gaseous exchange occurs across the respiratory membrane in the alveolar duct and in the millions of alveoli.

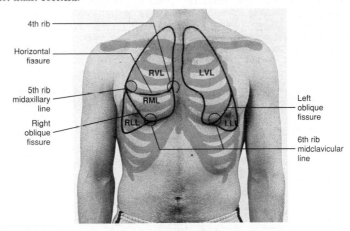

4th rib

Horizontal
fissure

RVL   LVL

5th rib
midaxillary
line

RML

Left
oblique
fissure

Right
oblique
fissure

RLL   LLL

6th rib
midclavicular
line

▶ Figure 11–3   Lobes of the lungs—anterior

In the anterior chest, the *apex*, or highest point, of lung tissue is 3 or 4 cm above the inner third of the clavicles (Fig. 11–3). The *base*, or lower border, rests on the dia-phragm. The right lung has three lobes, and the left lung has two lobes. The lobes are separated by fissures.

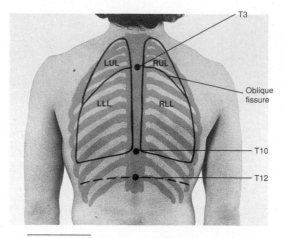

▶ Figure 11–4   Lobes of the lungs—posterior

Posteriorly, the location of the seventh cervical vertebra (C7) marks the apex of lung tissue and T10 usually corresponds to the base (Fig. 11–4). The most remarkable point about the posterior chest is that it is almost all lower lobe. The upper lobes occupy only a small band of tissue from the apices down to T3 or T4. The rest is all lower lobe. The right middle lobe does not project onto the posterior chest at all.

TRANSCULTURAL CONSIDERATIONS

Biocultural differences occur in the size of the thoracic cavity. In descending order, the largest chest volumes are found in whites, blacks, Asians, and Native Americans. Even considering the shorter height of Asians, their chest volume remains significantly lower than in whites and blacks.

SUBJECTIVE DATA

Cough (duration, productive of sputum)

Shortness of breath (with what activity)

Chest pain with breathing

Past history of respiratory disease (bronchitis, emphysema, asthma, pneumonia, tuberculosis)

Cigarette smoking (number of packs per day, number of years smoked)

Environmental exposure that affects breathing

Self-care behaviors (last Tb skin test, chest x-ray, influenza immunization)

OBJECTIVE DATA

Equipment Needed

Stethoscope

Small ruler marked in centimeters

Marking pen

Preparation

Ask the person to sit upright and the male to disrobe to the waist. Leave the gown on the female open at the back.

· METHOD OF EXAMINATION

NORMAL RANGE OF FINDINGS	ABNORMAL FINDINGS

THE POSTERIOR CHEST

Inspect the Posterior Chest

Shape and configuration. The spinous processes are in a straight line. The thorax is symmetric with downward sloping ribs. The scapulae are placed symmetrically.

Skeletal deformities may limit thoracic cage excursions: scoliosis, kyphosis (see Table 15–2, pp. 175).

The anteroposterior diameter of the chest is less than the transverse diameter. The ratio of anteroposterior: transverse diameter is from 1:2 to 5:7.

The neck muscles and trapezius muscles are developed normally for age and occupation.

Anteroposterior = transverse diameter or "barrel chest" with ribs horizontal, occurs in chronic emphysema due to hyperinflation of the lungs.

Neck muscles are hypertrophied in chronic obstructive pulmonary disease (COPD) from aiding in forced respirations.

Position. This includes a relaxed posture with arms comfortably at the sides or in the lap.

With COPD, a tripod position (leaning forward with arms braced against knees, chair or bed) gives leverage so that the rectus abdominis, intercostal, and accessory neck muscles can aid in expiration.

Skin color and condition. Color should be consistent with person's genetic background, with no cyanosis or pallor. Note any lesions.

Palpate the Posterior Chest

Symmetric Expansion

Confirm *symmetric chest expansion* by placing your warmed hands on the posterolateral chest wall with thumbs at the level of T-9 or T-10. Slide your hands medially to pinch up a small fold of skin between your thumbs. Ask the person to take a deep breath; your thumbs should move apart symmetrically. Note any lag in expansion.

Unequal chest expansion occurs with marked atelectasis or pneumonia; with thoracic trauma, such as fractured ribs; or pneumothorax.

Pain accompanies deep breathing when the pleurae are inflamed.

NORMAL RANGE OF FINDINGS	ABNORMAL FINDINGS

Tactile Fremitus

Tactile fremitus is a palpable vibration. Use the palmar base (the ball) of the fingers of one hand and touch the person's chest while he or she repeats the words "ninety-nine" or "blue moon." Start over the lung apices and palpate from one side to another; the vibrations should feel the same in the corresponding area on each side.

Normally, fremitus is most prominent between the scapulae and around the sternum, sites where the major bronchi are closest to the chest wall. Fremitus normally decreases as you progress down because more and more tissue impedes sound transmission.

Decreased fremitus occurs when anything obstructs transmission of vibrations, e.g., obstructed bronchus, pleural effusion or thickening, pneumothorax, or emphysema.

Increased fremitus occurs with compression or consolidation of lung tissue, e.g., lobar pneumonia (see Table 15–7, p. 517 in Jarvis: *Physical Examination and Health Assessment*).

Chest Wall

Using the fingers, gently *palpate the entire chest* wall. Note any areas of tenderness, increased skin temperature and moisture, any superficial lumps or masses, and any skin lesions.

Crepitus is a coarse, crackling sensation palpable over the skin surface. It occurs in subcutaneous emphysema when air escapes from the lung and enters the subcutaneous tissue, as following open thoracic injury or surgery.

Percuss the Posterior Chest

Lung Fields

Start at the apices and percuss in the interspaces: make a side-to-side comparison all the way down the lung region. Percuss at 5-cm intervals. Avoid the scapulae and ribs.

Resonance predominates in healthy lung tissue in the adult. The resonant note may be modified somewhat in the athlete with a heavily muscular chest wall and in the heavily obese adult in whom subcutaneous fat produces scattered dullness.

Hyperresonance is found when too much air is present, as in emphysema or pneumothorax.

A *dull* note signals abnormal density in the lungs, as with pneumonia, pleural effusion, atelectasis, or tumor.

Diaphragmatic Excursion

Percuss to map out the lower lung border, both in expiration and inspi-

An abnormally high level of dullness on the chest wall, as

NORMAL RANGE OF FINDINGS	ABNORMAL FINDINGS

ration. Measure the difference. This *diaphragmatic excursion* should be equal bilaterally and measure about 3 to 5 cm in adults, although it may be up to 7 to 8 cm in well-conditioned people.

well as absence of excursion, occurs with pleural effusion or atelectasis of the lower lobes.

Auscultate the Posterior Chest

Breath Sounds

Instruct the person to breathe through the mouth a little bit deeper than usual. While standing behind the person, listen to the following lung areas—posterior from the apices at C-7 to the bases (around T-10), and laterally from the axillae down to the seventh or eighth rib. Use the side-to-side sequence illustrated in Figure 11–5. You should expect to hear three types of normal breath sounds: bronchial (sometimes called tracheal or tubular), broncho vesicular, and vesicular (see Table 11–1 on p. 114).

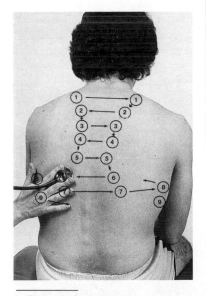

▶ Figure 11–5   Order of Auscultation

NORMAL RANGE OF FINDINGS	ABNORMAL FINDINGS

Note the normal location of the three types of breath sounds (Fig. 11–6 and Fig. 11–7 on p. 112).

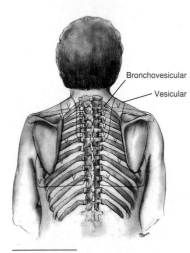

Bronchovesicular

Vesicular

▶ Figure 11–6   Breath sounds on the posterior chest

Adventitious Sounds

Note the presence of any *adventitious sounds*. These are abnormal sounds caused by moving air colliding with secretions in the tracheobronchial passageways or by the popping open of a previously deflated airway. Crackles (or rales) and wheezes (or rhonchi) are terms commonly used by many examiners (see Table 11–2 on pp. 114–115).

THE ANTERIOR CHEST

Inspect the Anterior Chest

Shape and configuration. The ribs are sloping downward with symmetric interspaces. The costal angle is within 90 degrees. Development of abdominal muscles is as expected for the person's age, weight, and athletic condition..

Facial expression. Relaxed and benign, indicating an unconscious effort of breathing

---

Decreased or absent breath sounds occur
1. When the bronchial tree is obstructed by secretions, mucous plug, or a foreign body.
2. In emphysema due to loss of elasticity in the lung fibers and decreased force of inspired air.
3. When anything obstructs transmission of sound, such as pleurisy or pleural thickening, or air (pneumothorax) or fluid (pleural effusion) in the pleural space.

Increased breath sounds— bronchial sounds are abnormal over the peripheral lung fields. They occur when consolidation (e.g., pneumonia) or compression yields a denser lung area that enhances the transmission of sound from the bronchi. When the inspired air reaches the alveoli, it hits solid lung tissue that conducts sound more efficiently to the surface.

Barrel chest has horizontal ribs and costal angle > 90 degrees.

Hypertrophy of abdominal muscles occurs with chronic emphysema.

Tense, strained, tired facies accompany COPD.

NORMAL RANGE OF FINDINGS	ABNORMAL FINDINGS

Level of consciousness. Alert and cooperative.

Cerebral hypoxia may be reflected by excessive drowsiness or by anxiety, restlessness, and irritability.

Skin color and condition. The lips and nailbeds are free of cyanosis or unusual pallor. The nails are of normal configuration.

Clubbing of distal phalanx occurs with chronic respiratory disease.

Quality of respirations. Normal, relaxed breathing is automatic and effortless, regular and even, and produces no noise. The chest expands symmetrically with each inspiration. Note any localized lag on inspiration.

Noisy breathing occurs with severe asthma or chronic bronchitis.

Unequal chest expansion occurs when part of the lung is obstructed or collapsed, as with pneumonia, or guarding to avoid postoperative incisional pain or the pain of pleurisy.

Rectus abdominis and internal intercostal muscles are used to force expiration in chronic obstructive pulmonary disease.

The respiratory rate is within normal limits for the person's age, and the pattern of breathing is regular. Occasional sighs normally punctuate breathing.

Tachypnea and hyperventilation, bradypnea and hypoventilation, periodic breathing (see Table 11–3 on p. 116).

Percuss the Anterior Chest

Begin at the apices. Percussing the interspaces and comparing one side to the other, move down the anterior chest.

Normally you hear a resonant note over healthy lung tissue. Note the borders of cardiac dullness normally found on the anterior chest and do not confuse these with suspected lung pathology. In the right hemithorax, the upper border of liver dullness is located in the fifth intercostal space in the right midclavicular line. On the left, tympany is evident over the gastric space (see Fig. 15–24, p. 503 in Jarvis: *Physical Examination and Health Assessment*).

Lungs are hyperinflated with chronic emphysema, resulting in hyperresonance where cardiac dullness would be expected.

Auscultate the Anterior Chest

Auscultate the lung fields over the anterior chest from the apices in the supraclavicular areas down to the sixth rib. Progress from side to

NORMAL RANGE OF FINDINGS	ABNORMAL FINDINGS

side as you move downward, and listen to one full respiration in each location. You should expect to hear vesicular breath sounds over most of the anterior lung fields as indicated in Figure 11–7.

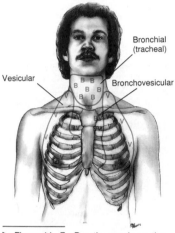

Vesicular

Bronchial (tracheal)

Bronchovesicular

▶ Figure 11–7   Breath sounds on the anterior chest

DEVELOPMENTAL CONSIDERATIONS
Infants and Children

Count the respiratory rate for 1 full minute, if possible when the infant is asleep, because infants reach rapid rates with very little excitation when awake. The respiratory pattern may be irregular when there are extremes in room temperature or with feeding or sleeping. Brief periods of apnea less than 10 or 15 seconds are common. This periodic breathing is more common in premature infants.

Auscultation normally yields bronchovesicular breath sounds in the peripheral lung fields in the infant and young child up to age 5 to 6, because of the relatively thin chest wall with underdeveloped musculature.

Rapid respiratory rates accompany pneumonia, fever, pain, heart disease, and anemia.

In an infant, tachypnea of 50 to 100 breaths per minute during sleep may be an early sign of left-sided congestive heart failure.

Periodic breathing with persistent or prolonged apnea (> 20 seconds) may signify an increased risk of sudden infant death syndrome (SIDS). Diminished breath sounds occur with pneumonia, atelectasis, pleural effusion, or pneumothorax.

NORMAL RANGE OF FINDINGS

ABNORMAL FINDINGS

Fine crackles are the adventitious sounds commonly heard in the immediate newborn period and are due to opening of the airways and clearing of fluid. Since the newborn's chest wall is so thin, transmission of sounds is enhanced and heard easily all over the chest, making localizations of breath sounds a problem. Even bowel sounds are easily heard in the chest. Try using the smaller pediatric diaphragm endpiece or place the bell over the infant's interspaces, not over the ribs.

Persistent fine crackles scattered over the chest occur with pneumonia, bronchiolitis, or atelectasis.

Crackles only in upper lung fields occur with cystic fibrosis; crackles only in lower lung fields occur with heart failure.

Expiratory wheezing occurs with asthma or bronchiolitis.

Persistent peristaltic sounds with diminished breath sounds on the same side may indicate diaphragmatic hernia.

Stridor is a high-pitched inspiratory crowing sound heard without the stethoscope, occurring with croup or acute epiglottitis.

The Pregnant Female

The thoracic cage may appear wider and the costal angle may feel wider than in the nonpregnant state. Respirations may be deeper, although this can be quantified only with pulmonary function tests.

The Aging Adult

The chest cage commonly shows an increased anteroposterior diameter, giving a round barrel shape and *kyphosis* or an outward curvature of the thoracic spine. The person compensates by holding the head extended and tilted back.

You may palpate marked bony prominences because of decreased subcutaneous fat. Chest expansion may be somewhat decreased although still symmetric. The costal cartilages become calcified with age, resulting in a less mobile thorax.

The older person may fatigue easily, especially during auscultation when deep mouth-breathing is required. Take care that this person does not hyperventilate and become dizzy. Allow brief rest periods or quiet breathing. If the person does feel faint, holding the breath for a few seconds will restore equilibrium.

Table 11-1 ▶ Characteristics of Normal Breath Sounds

	PITCH	AMPLITUDE	DURATION	QUALITY	NORMAL LOCATION
Bronchial (Tracheal)	High	Loud	Inspiration < expiration	Harsh, hollow, tubular	Trachea and larynx
Broncho-vesicular	Moderate	Moderate	Inspiration = expiration	Mixed	Over major bronchi where fewer alveoli are located: posterior, between scapulae especially on right; anterior, around upper sternum in first and second intercostal spaces
Vesicular	Low	Soft	Inspiration > expiration	Rustling like the sound of the wind in the trees.	Over peripheral lung fields where air flows through smaller bronchioles and alveoli

A B N O R M A L   F I N D I N G S

Table 11-2 ▶ Adventitious Sounds*

SOUND	DESCRIPTION	MECHANISM	CLINICAL EXAMPLE
(1)-DISCONTINUOUS SOUNDS			
Crackles—fine (rales, crepitations) *Inspiration Expiration*	Discontinuous, high-pitched, short, crackling, popping sounds heard during inspiration and are not cleared by coughing.	Inhaled air collides with previously deflated airways: airways suddenly pop open, creating crackling sound.	*Late inspiratory crackles* occur with restrictive disease: pneumonia, congestive heart failure, and interstitial fibrosis. *Early inspiratory crackles* occur with obstructive disease: chronic bronchitis, asthma, and emphysema.

Table 11-2 ▶ Adventitious Sounds *Continued*

SOUND	DESCRIPTION	MECHANISM	CLINICAL EXAMPLE
(1)-DISCONTINUOUS SOUNDS			
Crackles—coarse (coarse rales)	Loud, low-pitched, bubbling, and gurgling sounds that start in early inspiration and may be present in expiration.	Inhaled air collides with secretions in the trachea and large bronchi.	Pulmonary edema, pneumonia, pulmonary fibrosis, and in the terminally ill who have a depressed cough reflex.
Atelectatic crackles (atelectatic rales)	Sound like fine crackles but do not last and are not pathologic. Disappear after the first few breaths. Heard in axillae and bases (usually dependent) of lungs.	When sections of alveoli are not fully aerated, they deflate and accumulate secretions. Crackles are heard when these sections re-expand with a few deep breaths.	In aging adults, bedridden persons, or in persons just roused from sleep
Pleural friction rub	A very superficial sound that is coarse and low pitched; it has a grating quality as if two pieces of leather are being rubbed together. Sounds just like crackles, but *close* to the ear.	Caused when pleurae become inflamed and lose their normal lubricating fluid. Their opposing, roughened, pleural surfaces rub together during respiration.	Pleuritis accompanied by pain with breathing. (Rub disappears after a few days if pleural fluid accumulates and separates pleurae.)
(2)-CONTINUOUS SOUNDS			
Wheeze—high-pitched (sibilant rhonchi)	High-pitched, musical, squeaking sounds that predominate in expiration but may occur in both expiration and inspiration.	Air squeezed or compressed through passageways narrowed almost to closure by collapsing, swelling, secretions, or tumors.	Obstructive lung disease such as asthma or emphysema.
Wheeze—low-pitched (sonorous rhonchi)	Low-pitched, musical snoring, moaning sounds. They are heard throughout the cycle, although they are more prominent on expiration. May clear somewhat by coughing.	Airflow obstruction. The pitch of the wheeze cannot be correlated to the size of the passageway that generates it.	Bronchitis

* Although nothing in clinical practice seems to differ more than the nomenclature of adventitious sounds, most authorities concur on two categories: (1) discontinuous, discrete crackling sounds, and (2) continuous coarse, or musical sounds.

Table 11-3 ▶ Respiratory Patterns*

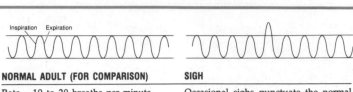

Inspiration Expiration

NORMAL ADULT (FOR COMPARISON)

Rate—10 to 20 breaths per minute
Depth—500 to 800 ml
Pattern—even
The ratio of pulse to respirations is fairly constant, about 4:1. Both values increase as a normal response to exercise, fear, or fever.

SIGH

Occasional sighs punctuate the normal breathing pattern and expand alveoli. Frequent sighs may indicate emotional dysfunction and may lead to hyperventilation and dizziness.

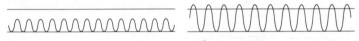

TACHYPNEA

Rapid shallow breathing. Increased rate >24 per minute. This is a normal response to fever, fear, or exercise. Rate also increases with respiratory insufficiency, pneumonia, alkalosis, pleurisy, and lesions in the pons.

HYPERVENTILATION

Increase in both rate and depth. Normally occurs with extreme exertion, fear, or anxiety. Also occurs with diabetic ketoacidosis (Kussmaul's respirations), hepatic coma, salicylate overdose, lesions of the midbrain, and alteration in blood gas concentration.

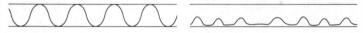

BRADYPNEA

Slow breathing. A decreased but regular rate (less than 10 per minute), as in drug-induced depression of the respiratory center in the medulla, increased intracranial pressure, and diabetic coma.

HYPOVENTILATION

An irregular, shallow pattern caused by an overdose of narcotics or anesthetics and with prolonged bedrest or conscious splinting of the chest to avoid respiratory pain.

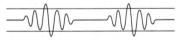

CHEYNE-STOKES RESPIRATION

A cycle in which respirations gradually increase in rate and depth and then decrease. The breathing periods last 30 to 45 seconds with periods of apnea (20 seconds) alternating the cycle. The most common cause is severe congestive heart failure; other causes are renal failure, meningitis, drug overdose, increased intracranial pressure. Occurs normally in infants and aging persons during sleep.

BIOT'S RESPIRATION

Similar to Cheyne-Stokes respiration except that pattern is irregular. A series of normal respirations (3 to 4) is followed by a period of apnea. The cycle length is variable, lasting anywhere from 10 seconds to 1 minute. Seen with head trauma, brain abscess, heat stroke, spinal meningitis, and encephalitis.

* Assess the (1) rate, (2) depth (tidal volume), and (3) pattern

☑ SUMMARY CHECKLIST

1 ▶ Inspection
   Thoracic cage
   Respirations
   Skin color and condition
   Person's position
   Facial expression
   Level of consciousness
2 ▶ Palpation
   Confirm symmetric expansion
   Tactile fremitus

Detect any lumps, masses, tenderness
3 ▶ Percussion
   Percuss over lung fields
   Estimate diaphragmatic excursion
4 ▶ Auscultation
   Assess normal breath sounds
   Note any abnormal breath sounds
   Note any adventitious sounds

Nursing Diagnoses Commonly Associated with the Thorax and Lungs — Respiratory Disorders

Activity intolerance

Anxiety

Ineffective airway clearance

Ineffective breathing pattern

Impaired gas exchange

Fatigue

Fluid volume excess

Potential for infection

Altered role performance

Self-care deficit

Altered tissue perfusion

Impaired home maintenance management

Pain

Sleep pattern disturbance

CHAPTER

12 Heart and Neck Vessels

The *precordium* is the area on the anterior chest overlying the heart and great vessels. The heart extends from the second to the fifth intercostal space, and from the right border of the sternum to the left midclavicular line (Fig. 12–1).

Think of the heart as an upside down triangle in the chest. The "top" of the heart is the broader *base*, and the bottom is the *apex*, which points down and to the left. During contraction, the apex beats against the chest wall, producing an *apical impulse.*

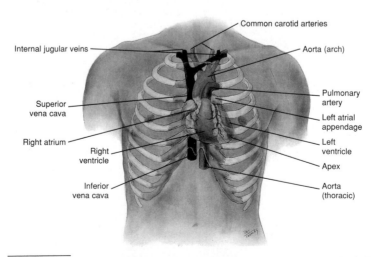

Internal jugular veins

Common carotid arteries

Aorta (arch)

Superior vena cava

Pulmonary artery

Left atrial appendage

Right atrium

Left ventricle

Right ventricle

Apex

Inferior vena cava

Aorta (thoracic)

▶ Figure 12–1 Position of the heart and great vessels

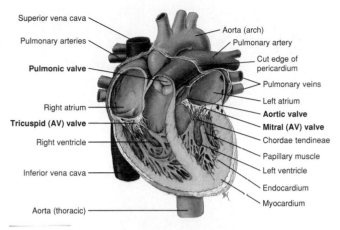

▶ Figure 12–2 Heart wall, chambers, and valves

The right side of the heart pumps blood into the lungs, and the left side of the heart simultaneously pumps blood into the body. Each side has an *atrium* and a *ventricle* (Fig. 12–2). The atrium is a thin-walled reservoir for holding blood, and the thick-walled ventricle is the muscular pumping chamber.

There are four valves in the heart. The two *atrioventricular* (AV) valves separate the atria and the ventricles. The right AV valve is the *tricuspid,* the left AV valve is the *bicuspid* or *mitral* valve. The AV valves open during the heart's filling phase, or *diastole,* to allow the ventricles to fill with blood.

The *semilunar* (SL) valves are set between the ventricles and the arteries. The SL valves are the *pulmonic* valve in the right side of the heart and the *aortic* valve in the left side of the heart. They open during pumping, or *systole,* to allow blood to be ejected from the heart.

Cardiovascular assessment includes the neck vessels—the carotid artery and the jugular veins (Fig. 12–3).

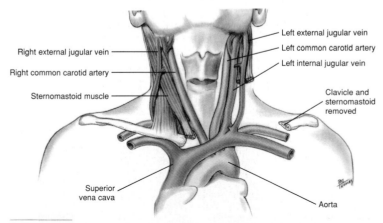

▶ Figure 12–3 Neck vessels—the carotid artery and the jugular veins

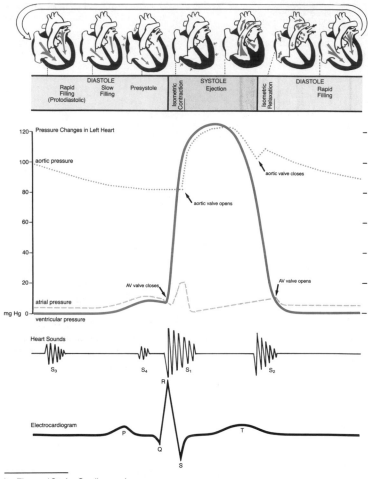

▶ Figure 12-4 Cardiac cycle

The rhythmic movement of blood through the heart is the *cardiac cycle*. It has two phases, *diastole* and *systole* (Fig. 12-4).

In *diastole*, the ventricles relax and fill with blood. The AV valves, the tricuspid and mitral, are open. During the first rapid filling phase, *proto-diastolic filling*, blood pours rapidly from the atria into the ventricles. Toward the end of diastole, the atria contract and push the last amount of blood into the ventricles, called *presystole*.

The closure of the AV valves contributes to the first heart sound (S_1) and signals the beginning of *systole*. The AV valves close to prevent any regurgitation of blood back up into the atria during contraction. Then the semilunar valves, the aortic and pulmonic, open and blood is ejected rapidly into the arteries.

After the ventricles' contents are ejected, the semilunar valves close. This causes the second heart sound (S_2) and signals the end of systole.

TRANSCULTURAL CONSIDERATIONS

Heart disease and stroke account for more than one-third of all deaths among individuals from culturally diverse backgrounds. Under age 35, heart disease mortality for Native Americans is approximately twice as high as that for all other Americans. Black men are nearly twice as likely to die from stroke as white men, and their death rate from stroke is more than double that of other ethnic groups.

Blacks, Puerto Ricans, Cubans, and Mexicans have a higher incidence of hypertension than whites. The prevalence of hypertension in blacks is 1.4 times greater than in whites despite a decline in mean blood pressure in blacks between 1960 and 1980 (Office of Minority Health, 1990).

SUBJECTIVE DATA

Chest pain

Dyspnea

Orthopnea

Cough

Fatigue

Cyanosis or pallor

Edema

Nocturia

Past history (hypertension, elevated cholesterol, heart murmur, rheumatic fever, anemia, heart disease)

Family history (hypertension, obesity, diabetes, coronary artery disease)

Personal habits (diet high in cholesterol, calories, salt; smoking; alcohol use; drugs; amount exercise)

OBJECTIVE DATA

Equipment Needed

Marking pen

Small centimeter ruler

Stethoscope with diaphragm and bell endpieces

Preparation

To evaluate the carotid arteries, the person can be sitting up. To assess the jugular veins and the precordium, the person should be supine with the head and chest slightly elevated. Stand on the person's right side.

METHOD OF EXAMINATION

NORMAL RANGE OF FINDINGS	ABNORMAL FINDINGS

THE NECK VESSELS

The Carotid Arteries

Palpate the Carotid Artery

Palpate gently and palpate only one carotid artery at a time to avoid compromising arterial blood to the brain.

Feel the contour and amplitude of the pulse. Normally the contour is smooth with a rapid upstroke and slower downstroke, and the normal strength is 2+ or moderate (see Chapter 14) and equal bilaterally.

Diminished pulse feels small and weak; occurs with decreased stroke volume.

Increased pulse feels full and strong; occurs with hyperkinetic states (see Table 14–1, p. 155).

Auscultate the Carotid Artery

For persons older than middle age or who show symptoms or signs of cardiovascular disease, auscultate each carotid artery for the presence of a *bruit*. This is a blowing, swishing sound indicating blood flow turbulence; normally there is none. Ask the person to hold his or her breath while you listen.

A bruit indicates turbulence due to a local vascular cause, e.g., atherosclerotic narrowing.

A murmur sounds much the same but is caused by a cardiac disorder. Some aortic valve murmurs radiate to the neck and must be distinguished from a local bruit.

The Jugular Veins

Inspect the Jugular Venous Pulse

Position the person supine with the torso elevated anywhere from a 30- to a 45-degree angle. Remove the pillow to avoid flexing the neck. Turn the person's head slightly away from the examined side, and direct a strong light tangentially onto the neck to highlight pulsations and shadows.

Note the external jugular veins overlying the sternomastoid muscle. In some persons, the veins are not visible at all; whereas, in others, they are full in the supine position. As the person is raised to a sitting position, these external jugulars flatten and disappear, usually at 45 degrees.

Unilateral distention of external jugular veins is due to local cause, e.g., kinking or aneurysm.

Full distended external jugular veins above 45 degrees signify increased central venous pressure (CVP).

NORMAL RANGE OF FINDINGS	ABNORMAL FINDINGS

THE PRECORDIUM

Inspection
Inspect the anterior chest

You may or may not see the *apical impulse*. When visible, it occupies the fourth or fifth intercostal space, at or inside the midclavicular line. It is easier to see in children or those with thinner chest walls.

A *heave* or *lift* is a sustained forceful thrusting of the ventricle during systole. It occurs with ventricular hypertrophy and is seen at the sternal border or the apex.

Palpation
Palpate the Apical Impulse

(This used to be called the point of maximal impulse or PMI).

Localize the apical impulse precisely using one finger pad.

Note

- Location—the apical impulse should occupy only one interspace, the fourth or fifth, and be at or medial to the midclavicular line.
- Size—normally 1 cm × 2 cm
- Amplitude—normally a short, gentle tap.
- Duration—short, normally occupies only first half of systole.

Cardiac enlargement:

- Left ventricular dilatation (volume overload) displaces apical impulse down and to the left and increases size more than 1 space.
- Increased force and duration but no change in location occurs with left ventricular hypertrophy and no dilatation (pressure overload).

The apical impulse is palpable in about half of adults. It is not palpable with obese persons or persons with thick chest walls. With high cardiac output states (anxiety, fever, hyperthyroidism, anemia), the apical impulse increases in amplitude and duration.

Apical impulse is not palpable with pulmonary emphysema due to overriding lungs.

Palpate Across the Precordium

Using the palmar aspects of your four fingers, gently palpate the apex, the left sternal border, and the base, searching for any other pulsations; normally there are none. If any are present, note the timing. Use the carotid artery pulsation as a guide or auscultate as you palpate.

A *thrill* is a palpable vibration. It feels like the throat of a purring cat. The thrill signifies turbulent blood flow and accompanies loud murmurs. Absence of a thrill, however, does not necessarily rule out the presence of a murmur.

NORMAL RANGE OF FINDINGS	ABNORMAL FINDINGS

Auscultation

Auscultate the Heart Sounds

Identify the auscultatory areas where you will listen. The four traditional valve "areas" (Fig. 12–5) are not over the actual anatomic locations of the valves but are the sites on the chest wall where sounds produced by the valves are best heard:

- Second right interspace—Aortic valve area.
- Second left interspace—Pulmonic valve area.
- Left lower sternal border—Tricuspid valve area.
- Fifth interspace at around left midclavicular line—Mitral valve area.

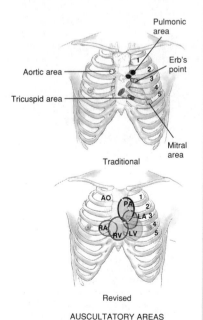

AUSCULTATORY AREAS

▶ Figure 12–5

NORMAL RANGE OF FINDINGS

ABNORMAL FINDINGS

Do not limit your auscultation to only four locations because sounds produced by the valves may be heard all over the precordium. Learn to inch your stethoscope in a "Z" pattern, from the base of the heart across and down, then over to the apex; or, start at the apex and work your way up. Include the sites shown in Figure 12–5.

Begin with the diaphragm endpiece and use the following routine: (1) Note the rate and rhythm, (2) identify S_1 and S_2, (3) assess S_1 and S_2 separately, (4) listen for extra heart sounds, and (5) listen for murmurs.

Note the rate and rhythm. The rate changes normally from 60 to 100 beats per minute. The rhythm should be regular, although *sinus arrhythmia* occurs normally in young adults and children. With sinus arrhythmia, the rhythm varies with the person's breathing, increasing at the peak of inspiration, and slowing with expiration. Note any other irregular rhythm.

Premature beat—an isolated beat is early or a pattern occurs in which every third or fourth beat sounds early.

Irregularly-irregular—no pattern to the sounds; beats come rapidly and at random intervals.

Identify S_1 and S_2. Usually, you can identify S_1 instantly because you hear a pair of sounds close to others (lubb dupp), and S_1 is the first of the pair. Other guidelines to distinguish S_1 from S_2 are:

- S_1 is louder than S_2 at the apex; S_2 is louder than S_1 at the base.
- S_1 coincides with the carotid artery pulsation.
- S_1 coincides with the R wave (the upstroke of the QRS complex) if the person is on an ECG monitor.

Listen to S_1 and S_2 separately. Note whether each heart sound is normal, accentuated, diminished, or split. Inch your diaphragm across the chest as you do this.

Causes of accentuated or diminished S_1 (see Table 16–2, p. 571 in Jarvis: *Physical Examination and Health Assessment*).

Both heart sounds are diminished with conditions that place an increased amount of tissue between the heart and your stethoscope: emphysema (hyperinflated lungs), obesity, pericardial fluid.

NORMAL RANGE OF FINDINGS   ABNORMAL FINDINGS

First Heart Sound (S₁). Caused by closure of the AV valves, S_1 signals the beginning of systole. You can hear it over the entire precordium, though it is loudest at the apex (Fig. 12–6).

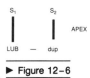

► Figure 12–6

Second Heart Sound (S₂). S_2 is associated with closure of the semilunar valves. You can hear it with the diaphragm, over the entire precordium, though S_2 is loudest at the base (Fig. 12–7).

► Figure 12–7

Splitting of S₂. A split S_2 is a normal phenomenon that occurs toward the end of inspiration in some people. Recall that closure of the aortic and pulmonic valves is nearly synchronous. Because of the effects of respiration on the heart, inspiration separates the timing of the two valves' closure, and the aortic valve closes 0.06 seconds before the pulmonic valve. Instead of one DUPP, you hear a split sound—T-DUPP (Fig. 12–8). During expiration, synchrony returns and the aortic and pulmonic components fuse together. A split S_2 is heard only in the pulmonic valve area, the second left interspace.

Accentuated or diminished S_2 (see Table 16–3, p. 572 in Jarvis: *Physical Examination and Health Assessment*).

NORMAL RANGE OF FINDINGS   ABNORMAL FINDINGS

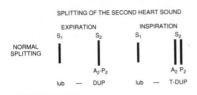

▶ Figure 12-8

Concentrate on the split as you watch the person's chest rise up and down with breathing. The split S_2 occurs about every fourth heartbeat, fading in with inhalation and fading out with exhalation.

Focus on systole, then on diastole, and listen for any *extra heart sounds*. Listen with the diaphragm, then switch to the bell, covering all auscultatory areas. Usually, these are silent periods. When you do detect an extra heart sound, listen carefully to note its timing and characteristics. During systole, the midsystolic click is the most common extra sound. The third heart sound and fourth heart sound occur in diastole; either may be normal or abnormal (see Table 12-1, page 133).

Listen for murmurs. A murmur is a blowing, swooshing sound that occurs with turbulent blood flow in the heart or great vessels. If you hear a murmur, describe it by indicating these characteristics:

Timing—Systole or diastole.

Loudness—The intensity in terms of six "grades."
Grade I—barely audible, heard only in a quiet room and then with difficulty
Grade II—clearly audible, but faint
Grade III—moderately loud
Grade IV—loud, associated with a thrill palpable on the chest wall
Grade V—very loud, heard with one corner of the stethoscope lifted off the chest wall

A fixed split is unaffected by respiration; the split is always there.

A paradoxical split is the opposite of what you would expect; the sounds fuse on inspiration and split on expiration (see Table 16-4, pp. 572-573 in Jarvis: *Physical Examination and Health Assessment*).

For a description of pathologic murmurs, using these characteristics, see Table 16-9, pp. 580-583, in Jarvis: *Physical Examination and Health Assessment*.

NORMAL RANGE OF FINDINGS   ABNORMAL FINDINGS

Grade VI—loudest, still heard with entire stethoscope lifted just off the chest wall

Pitch—High, medium, or low.

Pattern—Growing louder (crescendo), tapering off (decrescendo), or increasing to a peak and then decreasing (crescendo-decrescendo, or diamond-shaped). Since the entire murmur is just milliseconds long, it takes practice to diagnose pattern.

Quality—Musical, blowing, harsh, or rumbling.

Location—Area of maximum intensity of the murmur (where it is best heard) as noted by the valve area or intercostal spaces.

Radiation—Heard in another place on the precordium, the neck, the back, or the axilla.

Posture—Murmurs may disappear or be enhanced by a change in position.

Some murmurs are common in healthy children or adolescents and are termed *innocent* or *functional*. The contractile force of the heart is greater in children. This increases blood flow velocity. The increased velocity plus a smaller chest measurement makes an audible murmur. The innocent murmur is generally soft (Grade II), midsystolic, short, crescendo-decrescendo, and with a vibratory or musical quality ("vooot" sound like fiddle strings). Also, the innocent murmur is heard at the second or third left intercostal space and disappears with sitting, and the young person has no associated signs of cardiac dysfunction.

Although it is important to distinguish innocent murmurs from pathologic ones, it is best to suspect all murmurs as pathologic until proved otherwise. Diagnostic tests such as ECG, phonocardiogram, and echocardiogram are needed to establish an accurate diagnosis.

NORMAL RANGE OF FINDINGS	ABNORMAL FINDINGS

Change position. After auscultating in the supine position, roll the person toward his or her left side. Listen with the bell at the apex for the presence of any diastolic filling sounds.

S_3 and S_4, and the murmur of mitral stenosis may sometimes be heard only when on the left side.

DEVELOPMENTAL CONSIDERATIONS

Infants

Auscultate using the small (pediatric size) diaphragm and bell. The heart rate may range from 100 to 180 per minute immediately after birth, then stabilize to an average of 120 to 140 per minute. Infants normally have wide fluctuations with activity, from 170 per minute or more with crying or being active to 70 to 90 per minute with sleeping.

Expect the heart rhythm to have sinus arrhythmia, the phasic speeding up or slowing down with the respiratory cycle.

Rapid rates make it more challenging to evaluate heart sounds. Expect heart sounds to be louder in infants than in adults because of the infant's thinner chest wall. Splitting of S_2 just after the height of inspiration is common, not at birth but beginning a few hours after birth.

Murmurs in the immediate newborn period do not necessarily indicate congenital heart disease. Murmurs are relatively common in the first 2 to 3 days because of fetal shunt closure. These murmurs are usually Grade I or II, systolic, accompany no other signs of cardiac disease, and disappear in 2 to 3 days. The murmur of patent ductus arteriosus (PDA) is a continuous machinery murmur, which disappears by 2 to 3 days.

On the other hand, absence of a murmur in the immediate newborn period does not ensure a perfect heart; congenital defects can be present that are not signaled by an early murmur. It is best to listen fre-

Persistent tachycardia,

- >200 per minute in newborns or
- >150 per minute in infants

Bradycardia

- <90 per minute—all warrant further investigation

Investigate any irregularity except sinus arrhythmia.

Fixed split S_2 occurs with the murmur of atrial septal defect (ASD).

Persistent murmur after 2 to 3 days, holosystolic murmurs or those that last into diastole, and those that are loud all warrant further evaluation.

For more information on murmurs due to congenital heart defects, see Table 16–8, pp. 578–579 in Jarvis: *Physical Examination and Health Assessment.*

NORMAL RANGE OF FINDINGS	ABNORMAL FINDINGS

quently and to note and describe any murmur according to the characteristics listed on p. 127–128.

Children

Note any extracardiac or cardiac signs that may indicate heart disease; normally there are none.

Signs that indicate heart disease include: poor weight gain, developmental delay, persistent tachycardia, tachypnea, dyspnea on exertion, cyanosis, and clubbing. Note that clubbing of fingers and toes usually does not appear until late in the first year, even with severe cyanotic defects.
Note any obvious bulge or any heave—these are not normal.

The apical impulse is sometimes visible in children with thin chest walls.

Palpate the apical impulse: in the fourth intercostal space to the left of the midclavicular line until age 4; at the fourth interspace at the midclavicular line from age 4 to age 6; and in the fifth interspace to the right of the midclavicular line at age 7.

The average heart rate slows as the child grows older, although it is still variable with rest or activity.

The heart rhythm remains characterized by sinus arrhythmia. Physiologic S_3 is common in children (see Table 12–1). It occurs in early diastole, just after S_2, and is a dull, soft sound best heard at the apex.

Heart murmurs that are innocent (or functional) in origin are very common through childhood. Most innocent murmurs have these characteristics: soft, relatively short, systolic ejection murmur; medium pitch; vibratory; best heard at the left lower sternal or midsternal border, with no radiation to the apex, base, or back.

The apical impulse moves laterally with cardiac enlargement.
Thrill, a palpable vibration.

The Pregnant Female

The vital signs usually yield an increase in resting pulse rate of 10 to 15 beats per minute and a drop in blood pressure from the normal prepregnancy level. Blood pressure decreases to its lowest point during the

Suspect pregnancy-induced hypertension with a sustained rise of 30 mmHg systolic or 15 mmHg diastolic under basal conditions.

NORMAL RANGE OF FINDINGS	ABNORMAL FINDINGS

second trimester and then slowly rises during the third trimester. Blood pressure varies with position. It is usually lowest in the left lateral recumbent position, a bit higher when supine (except for some who experience hypotension when supine), and highest when sitting.

Palpation of the apical impulse is higher and lateral as compared with the normal position, as the enlarging uterus elevates the diaphragm and displaces the heart up and to the left and rotates it on its long axis.

Auscultation of the heart sounds shows changes due to the increased blood volume and workload:

Heart sounds

- exaggerated splitting of S_1 and increased loudness of S_1
- a loud, easily heard S_3

Heart murmurs

- a systolic murmur in 90 percent, which disappears soon after delivery
- a soft, diastolic murmur heard transiently in 19 percent
- a continuous murmur arising from breast vasculature in 10 percent, the *mammary souffle*, (pronounced SOOF'f'l) (Cutforth and MacDonald, 1966).

The Aging Adult

A gradual rise in systolic blood pressure is common with aging; the diastolic blood pressure stays fairly constant with a resulting widening of pulse pressure. Some older adults experience *orthostatic hypotension*, a sudden drop in blood pressure when rising to sit or stand.

The chest often increases in anteroposterior diameter with aging. This makes it more difficult to palpate the apical impulse and to hear the splitting of S_2. The S_4 often occurs in older people with no known cardiac disease.

NORMAL RANGE OF FINDINGS   ABNORMAL FINDINGS

Occasional ectopic beats are common and do not necessarily indicate underlying heart disease. When in doubt, obtain an ECG; however, consider that the ECG only records for one isolated minute in time and may need to be supplemented by 24-hour ambulatory heart monitoring.

Table 12-1 ▶ Diastolic Extra Sounds

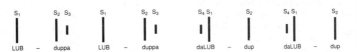

THIRD HEART SOUND

The S_3 is a ventricular filling sound. It occurs in early diastole during the rapid filling phase. Your hearing quickly accommodates to the S_3, so it is best heard when you listen initially. It sounds after S_2, is a dull, soft sound, and it is low pitched, like "distant thunder." It is heard best in a quiet room, at the apex, with the bell held tightly (just enough to form a seal), and with the person in the left lateral position.

The S_3 can be confused with a split S_2. Use these guidelines to distinguish the S_3:

- Location—the S_3 is heard at the apex or left lower sternal border; the split S_2 at the base.
- Respiratory variation—the S_3 does not vary in timing with respirations; the split S_2 does.
- Pitch—the S_3 is lower pitched; the pitch of the split S_2 stays the same.

The S_3 may be normal (physiologic) or abnormal (pathologic). The *physiologic* S_3 is heard frequently in children and young adults; it occasionally may persist after age 40, especially in women. The normal S_3 usually disappears when the person sits up.

In adults, the S_3 is usually abnormal. The *pathologic* S_3 is also called a *ventricular gallop* or an S_3 *gallop*, and it persists when sitting up. The S_3 indicates decreased compliance of the ventricles, as in congestive heart failure. The S_3 may be the earliest sign of heart failure.

The S_3 is also found in high cardiac output states in the absence of heart disease, such as hyperthyroidism, anemia, and pregnancy. When the primary condition is corrected, the gallop disappears.

FOURTH HEART SOUND

S_4 is a ventricular filling sound. It occurs when the atria contract late in diastole. It is heard immediately before S_1. This is a very soft sound, of very low pitch. You need a good bell, and you must listen for it. It is heard best at the apex, with the person in left lateral position.

A *physiologic* S_4 may occur in adults older than 40 or 50 with no evidence of cardiovascular disease, especially after exercise.

A *pathologic* S_4 is termed an *atrial gallop* or an S_4 *gallop*. It occurs with decreased compliance of the ventricle, e.g., coronary artery disease, cardiomyopathy, and with systolic overload (afterload), including outflow obstruction to the ventricle (aortic stenosis) and systemic hypertension.

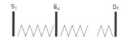

PERICARDIAL FRICTION RUB

Inflammation of the precordium gives rise to a friction rub. The sound is high pitched and scratchy, like sandpaper being rubbed. It is best heard with the diaphragm, with the person sitting up and leaning forward, and with the breath held in expiration.

A friction rub can be heard any place on the precordium but is usually best heard at the apex and left lower sternal border, places where the pericardium comes in close contact with the chest wall. Timing may be systolic and diastolic.

The friction rub of pericarditis is common during the first week following a myocardial infarction and may last only a few hours.

☑ SUMMARY CHECKLIST

Cardiovascular Examination
1 ▶ Neck
   A. Carotid pulse—observe and palpate
   B. Observe jugular venous pulse
   C. Estimate jugular venous pressure
2 ▶ Precordium
   A. Inspection and palpation
     1. Describe location of apical impulse
     2. Note any heave (lift) or thrill
   B. Auscultation
     1. Identify anatomic areas where you listen

2. Note rate and rhythm of heartbeat
3. Identify S_1 and S_2 and note any variation
4. Listen in systole and diastole for any extra heart sounds
5. Listen in systole and diastole for any murmurs
6. Repeat sequence with bell
7. Listen at the apex with person in left lateral position

Nursing Diagnoses Commonly Associated with the Heart and Circulatory Disorders

Activity intolerance

Anxiety

Alteration in tissue perfusion

Decreased cardiac output

Dysfunctional grieving

Fear

Ineffective individual coping

Ineffective breathing pattern

Impaired home maintenance management

Pain

Potential for injury

Noncompliance

Powerlessness

Role performance, altered

Self-care deficit

Sexuality patterns, altered

Tissue perfusion, altered

CHAPTER

13 Abdomen

The abdomen is a large oval cavity extending from the diaphragm down to the brim of the pelvis (Fig. 13–1). For convenience in description, the abdominal wall is divided into four quadrants by an imaginary vertical and a horizontal line bisecting the umbilicus.

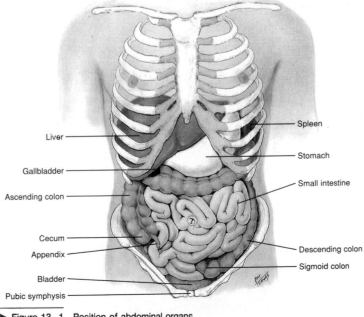

Liver
Gallbladder
Ascending colon
Cecum
Appendix
Bladder
Pubic symphysis

Spleen
Stomach
Small intestine
Descending colon
Sigmoid colon

▶ Figure 13–1   Position of abdominal organs

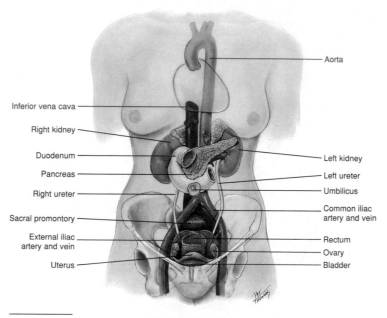

Aorta

Inferior vena cava

Right kidney

Duodenum

Pancreas

Right ureter

Sacral promontory

External iliac
artery and vein

Uterus

Left kidney

Left ureter

Umbilicus

Common iliac
artery and vein

Rectum

Ovary

Bladder

▶ Figure 13–2   Relationship of aorta to deep abdominal viscera

The aorta is just to the left of midline in the upper abdomen (Fig. 13–2). At 2 cm below the umbilicus, it bifurcates into the right and left iliac arteries.

The bean-shaped kidneys are retroperitoneal, or posterior to the abdominal contents.

SUBJECTIVE DATA

Change in appetite

Dysphagia (difficulty swallowing)

Food intolerance

Abdominal pain

Nausea/vomiting

Bowel habits

Rectal conditions

Past abdominal history (ulcer, gallbladder disease, hepatitis, appendicitis, colitis, hernia)

Medications (prescription, over-the-counter including antacids)

Alcohol, drug, cigarette use

Nutritional assessment (24-hour recall)

OBJECTIVE DATA

Equipment Needed

Stethoscope

Small centimeter ruler

Skin-marking pen

Preparation

Turn on a strong overhead light and a secondary stand light. Expose the abdomen so that it is fully visible. Drape the genitalia and female breasts.

The following measures will enhance abdominal wall relaxation:

- Empty the bladder, saving a urine specimen if needed.
- Keep the room warm.
- Position supine, with the head on a pillow, knees bent or on a pillow, and the arms at the sides or across the chest.
- Keep the stethoscope endpiece warm, your hands warm, and your fingernails very short.
- Examine any painful areas last to avoid any muscle guarding.
- Use distraction: breathing exercises, emotive imagery, your low, soothing voice, and the person relating his or her abdominal history while you palpate.

METHOD OF EXAMINATION

NORMAL RANGE OF FINDINGS	ABNORMAL FINDINGS
INSPECTION **Inspect Contour, Symmetry, Umbilicus, Skin, Pulsation or movement, and Hair Distribution.**	
Contour. Stand on the person's right side and stoop to gaze across the abdomen. Determine the profile from the rib margin to the pubic bone, normally flat to rounded.	Protuberant abdomen, abdominal distention (see Table 17–3, pp. 624–627 in Jarvis: *Physical Examination and Health Assessment*). Scaphoid abdomen occurs with malnourishment.
Symmetry. Shine a light across the abdomen toward you or shine it lengthwise across the person. The abdomen should be symmetric bilaterally. Note any localized bulging, visible mass, or asymmetric shape.	Bulges, masses. Hernia—protrusion of abdominal viscera through abnormal opening in muscle wall (see Table 17–4, pp. 627–628 in Jarvis: *Physical Examination and Health Assessment*).

NORMAL RANGE OF FINDINGS	ABNORMAL FINDINGS

Umbilicus. It is normally midline and inverted with no sign of discoloration, inflammation, or hernia. It becomes everted and pushed upward with pregnancy.

Everted with ascites or underlying mass.
Deeply sunken with obesity.
Enlarged and everted with umbilical hernia.

Skin. The surface is smooth and even, with homogeneous color.

Redness with localized inflammation.
Jaundice (shows best in natural daylight).
Skin glistening and taut occurs with ascites.
Cutaneous angiomas (spider nevi) occur with portal hypertension or liver disease.
Lesions, rashes (see Chapter 5).

There are normally no lesions, although sometimes well-healed surgical scars are present. If a scar is present, draw its location in the person's record, indicating the length in centimeters.

Pulsation or Movement. Pulsations from the aorta may show beneath the skin in the epigastric area, particularly in thin persons with good muscle wall relaxation. Respiratory movement also shows in the abdomen, particularly in males.

Marked pulsation of the aorta occurs with widened pulse pressure (e.g., hypertension, aortic insufficiency, thyrotoxicosis) and with aortic aneurysm.
Marked visible peristalsis, together with a distended abdomen, indicates intestinal obstruction.

Demeanor. A comfortable person is relaxed quietly on the examining table and has a benign facial expression and slow, even respirations.

Restlessness and constant turning to find a comfortable position occur with the colicky pain of gastroenteritis or bowel obstruction.
Absolute stillness, resisting any movement, is demonstrated with the pain of peritonitis.
Knees flexed up, facial grimacing, and rapid, uneven respirations also indicate pain.

AUSCULTATION

Auscultate Bowel Sounds and Vascular Sounds

This is done next because percussion and palpation can increase peristalsis which would give a false interpretation of bowel sounds. Use the diaphragm endpiece and hold the stethoscope lightly against the skin. Begin in the RLQ, at the ileocecal

NORMAL RANGE OF FINDINGS	ABNORMAL FINDINGS

valve area, because bowel sounds are normally always present here.

Bowel Sounds. Note the character and frequency, normally high-pitched, gurgling, cascading sounds, occurring irregularly anywhere from 5 to 30 times per minute. Do not both to count them. Judge if they are normal, hypoactive, or hyperactive.

Two distinct patterns of abnormal bowel sounds may occur:
1. *Hyperactive* sounds are loud, high-pitched, rushing, tinkling sounds that signal increased motility. They occur with early mechanical bowel obstruction, gastroenteritis, brisk diarrhea, laxative use, and subsiding paralytic ileus.
2. *Hypoactive* or *absent* sounds follow abdominal surgery or with inflammation of the peritoneum or from late bowel obstruction (see Table 17–5, pp. 628–629 in Jarvis: *Physical Examination and Health Assessment*).

Vascular Sounds. Note the presence of any vascular sounds or *bruits*. Using firmer pressure, check over the aorta, renal arteries, iliac and femoral arteries, especially in people with hypertension (Fig. 13–3). Usually, there is no such sound.

Note location, pitch, and timing of a vascular sound.

A systolic bruit is a pulsatile, blowing sound.

Venous hum.

Peritoneal friction rub (see Table 17–6, p. 630 in Jarvis: *Physical Examination and Health Assessment*).

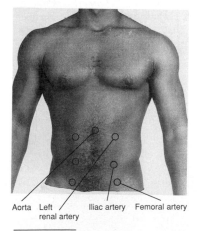

Aorta Left   Iliac artery   Femoral artery
       renal artery

▶ Figure 13–3 Sites to listen for vascular sounds

NORMAL RANGE OF FINDINGS	ABNORMAL FINDINGS

PERCUSSION

Percuss General Tympany, Liver Span, and Splenic Dullness

General Tympany. Percuss lightly in all four quadrants. Tympany should predominate because air in the intestines rises to the surface when the person is supine.

Dullness occurs over a distended bladder, adipose tissue, fluid, or a mass.

Hyperresonance is present with gaseous distention.

Liver Span. Measure the height of the liver in the right midclavicular line. Begin in the area of lung resonance and percuss down the interspaces until the sound changes to a dull quality. Mark the spot, usually in the fifth intercostal space. Then find abdominal tympany and percuss up in the midclavicular line. Mark where the sound changes from tympany to a dull sound, normally at the right costal margin.

Measure the distance between the two marks; the normal liver span in the adult ranges from 6 to 12 cm. Taller people have longer livers. Males also have a larger liver span than females of the same height. Overall, the mean liver span in 10.5 cm for males and 7 cm for females.

An enlarged liver span indicates liver enlargement or *hepatomegaly*.

Accurate detection of liver borders is confused by dullness above fifth intercostal space, which occurs with lung disease, e.g., pleural effusion or consolidation; lower border of dullness pushed up with ascites or pregnancy; gas distention in colon which obscures lower border.

Splenic Dullness. Locate it by a dull note from the 9th to 11th intercostal space just behind the left midaxillary line. The area of splenic dullness is normally not wider than 7 cm in the adult and should not encroach on the normal tympany over the gastric air bubble.

A dull note forward of the midaxillary line indicates enlargement of the spleen, as occurs with mononucleosis, trauma, and infection.

PALPATION

Palpate Surface and Deep Areas, Liver Edge, Spleen, and Kidneys

Light and Deep Palpation. Begin with light palpation. With the first four

Muscle guarding.
Rigidity.

NORMAL RANGE OF FINDINGS

ABNORMAL FINDINGS

fingers close together, depress the skin about 1 cm. Make a gentle rotary motion, lift the fingers (do not drag them) and move clockwise.

As you circle the abdomen, discriminate between voluntary muscle guarding and involuntary rigidity. Voluntary *guarding* occurs when the person is cold, tense, or ticklish. It is bilateral, and the muscles relax slightly during exhalation. Use relaxation measures to try to eliminate this type of guarding or it will interfere with deep palpation. If rigidity persists, it is probably involuntary.

Now perform **deep palpation**, pushing down about 5–8 cm (2–3 inches). Moving clockwise, explore the entire abdomen.

To overcome the resistance of a very large or obese abdomen, use a bimanual technique. Place your two hands on top of each other. The top hand does the pushing; the bottom hand is relaxed and can concentrate on the sense of palpation. With either technique, note the location, size, consistency, and mobility of any palpable organs and the presence of any abnormal enlargement, tenderness, or masses. Remember that some structures are normally palpable, as illustrated in Figure 13–4.

There is normally mild tenderness when palpating the sigmoid colon. Any other tenderness should be investigated.

If you identify a mass, first distinguish it from a normally palpable structure or an enlarged organ. Then note its:
1. Location
2. Size
3. Shape
4. Consistency (soft, firm, hard)
5. Surface (smooth, nodular)
6. Mobility (including movement with respirations)
7. Pulsatility
8. Tenderness

Large masses.
Tenderness

Involuntary *rigidity* is a constant, boardlike hardness of the muscles. It is a protective mechanism accompanying acute inflammation of the peritoneum. It may be unilateral, and the same area usually becomes painful when the person increases intra-abdominal pressure by attempting a sit-up.

Tenderness occurs with local inflammation, inflammation of the peritoneum or underlying organ, and with an enlarged organ whose capsule is stretched.

NORMAL RANGE OF FINDINGS	ABNORMAL FINDINGS

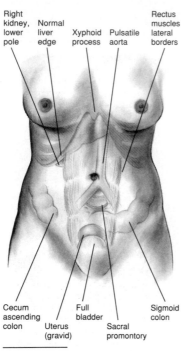

Right kidney, lower pole   Normal liver edge   Xyphoid process   Pulsatile aorta   Rectus muscles lateral borders

Cecum ascending colon   Uterus (gravid)   Full bladder   Sacral promontory   Sigmoid colon

▶ Figure 13–4   Normally palpable abdominal structures

Liver. Place your left hand under the person's back, parallel to the eleventh and 12th ribs, and lift up to support the abdominal contents. Place your right hand on the RUQ, with fingers parallel to the midline. (Fig. 13–5). Push deeply down and under the right costal margin. Ask the person to take a deep breath. It is normal to feel the edge of the liver bump your fingertips as the diaphragm pushes it down during inhalation. It feels like a firm, regular ridge. The liver is often not palpable and you may feel nothing firm.

Spleen. Normally, the spleen is not palpable and must be enlarged three times its normal size to be felt. Reach your left hand over the abdomen and behind the left side at the

Except with a depressed diaphragm, a liver palpated more than 1–2 cm below the right costal margin is considered enlarged. Record the number of centimeters it descends, and note its consistency (hard, nodular) and any tenderness.

NORMAL RANGE OF FINDINGS	ABNORMAL FINDINGS

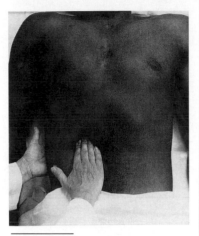

▶ Figure 13-5   Palpating the liver

eleventh and 12th ribs. Lift up for support. Place your right hand obliquely on the LUQ with the fingers pointing toward the left axilla and just inferior to the rib margin. Push your hand deeply down and under the left costal margin and ask the person to take a deep breath. You should feel nothing firm. When enlarged, the spleen slides out and bumps your fingertips.

The spleen enlarges with mononucleosis and trauma (see Table 17-7, pp. 630-632 in Jarvis: *Physical Examination and Health Assessment*). If you feel an enlarged spleen, do not continue to palpate it and refer the person. An enlarged spleen is friable and can rupture easily with overpalpation.

Describe the number of centimeters it extends below the left costal margin.

Kidneys. Search for the right kidney by placing your hands together in a "duckbill" position at the person's right flank. Press your two hands firmly and ask the person to take a deep breath. With most people, you will feel no change. Occasionally, you may feel the lower pole of the right kidney as a round, smooth mass slide between your fingers. Either condition is normal.

The left kidney sits 1 cm higher than the right kidney and is not normally palpable.

Enlarged kidney.
Kidney mass.

Aorta. Using your opposing thumb and fingers, palpate the aortic

NORMAL RANGE OF FINDINGS	ABNORMAL FINDINGS

pulsation in the upper abdomen slightly to the left of midline. It is normally 2.5–4 cm wide in the adult, and pulsates in an anterior direction.

Widened with aneurysm.

Prominent lateral pulsation with aortic aneurysm (see Table 17–7, pp. 630–632 in Jarvis: *Physical Examination and Health Assessment*).

Costovertebral Angle Tenderness. Place one hand over the 12th rib at the costovertebral angle on the back. Thump that hand with the ulnar edge of your other fist. The person normally feels a thud but no pain.

Sharp pain occurs with inflammation of the kidney or paranephric area.

Special Procedures

Rebound Tenderness. Choose a site away from the painful area. Hold your hand 90 degrees or perpendicular to the abdomen. Push down slowly and deeply; then lift up *quickly*. This makes structures that are indented by palpation rebound suddenly. A normal, or negative, response is absence of pain on release of pressure. Perform this test at the end of the examination because it can cause severe pain and muscle rigidity.

Pain on release of pressure confirms rebound tenderness, which is a reliable sign of peritoneal inflammation.

Fluid Wave For Ascites. Place the ulnar edge of another examiner's hand or the client's own hand firmly on the abdomen midline (Fig. 13–6). Place your left hand on the person's right flank. With your right hand, reach across the abdomen and

Acites occurs with congestive heart failure, portal hypertension, cirrhosis, hepatitis, pancreatitis, and cancer.

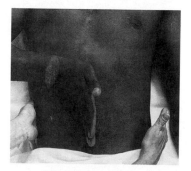

▶ Figure 13–6   Fluid wave

NORMAL RANGE OF FINDINGS	ABNORMAL FINDINGS

give the left flank a firm strike. If ascites is present, the blow will generate a fluid wave through the abdomen and you will feel a distinct tap on your left hand. If the abdomen is distended from gas or adipose tissue, you will feel no change.

A positive fluid wave test occurs with large amounts of ascitic fluid.

DEVELOPMENTAL CONSIDERATIONS

The Infant

The contour of the abdomen is protuberant because of the immature abdominal musculature. The skin contains a fine, superficial venous pattern. This may be visible in children up to the age of puberty.

Scaphoid shape.
Dilated veins.

The abdomen shows respiratory movement. The only other abdominal movement is occasional peristalsis which may be visible because of the thin musculature.

Marked peristalsis with pyloric stenosis.

Auscultation yields only bowel sounds, the metallic tinkling of peristalsis. There should be no vascular sounds.

Bruit.
Venous hum.

The Child

Under age 4 years, the abdomen looks protuberant when the child is both supine and standing. After age 4 years, the potbelly remains when standing because of lumbar lordosis, but the abdomen looks flat when supine. Normal movement on the abdomen includes respirations which remain abdominal until 7 years of age.

A scaphoid abdomen is associated with dehydration or malnutrition.

Under 7 years of age, the absence of abdominal respirations occurs with inflammation of the peritoneum.

The Aging Adult

On inspection, you may note increased deposits of subcutaneous fat on the abdomen and hips as it is redistributed away from the extremities. The abdominal musculature is thinner and has less tone than that

NORMAL RANGE OF FINDINGS	ABNORMAL FINDINGS

of the younger adult, so in the absence of obesity you may note peristalsis.

Owing to the thinner, softer abdominal wall, the organs may be easier to palpate (in the absence of obesity). The liver is easier to palpate. Normally, you will feel the liver edge at or just below the costal margin. With distended lungs and a depressed diaphragm, the liver is palpated lower, descending 1–2 cm below the costal margin with inhalation. The kidneys are easier to palpate.

Abdominal rigidity with acute abdominal conditions is less common in aging persons.

With an acute abdomen, the aging person often complains of less pain than would a younger person.

☑ SUMMARY CHECKLIST

1 ▶ Inspection
   Contour
   Symmetry
   Skin
   Pulsation or movement
   Demeanor
2 ▶ Auscultation
   Bowel sounds
   Note any vascular sounds

3 ▶ Percussion
   Percuss all four quadrants
   Percuss borders of liver, spleen
4 ▶ Palpation
   Light palpation in all four quadrants
   Deeper palpation in all four quadrants
   Palpate for liver, spleen, kidneys

Nursing Diagnoses Commonly Associated with Abdominal Disorders

Alteration in tissue perfusion: renal and gastrointestinal

Constipation

Perceived constipation

Colonic constipation

Diarrhea

Fluid volume deficit

Nutrition, altered: less than body requirements

Nutrition, altered: more than body requirements

Pain

Urinary retention

14 Peripheral Vascular System

The vascular system consists of the vessels in the body that transport fluid, such as blood or lymph.

The heart pumps blood through the *arteries* to all body tissues. The major artery to the leg is the *femoral*

artery, passing down under the inguinal ligament (Fig. 14–1).

Veins drain the blood from the tissues and return it to the heart (not illustrated).

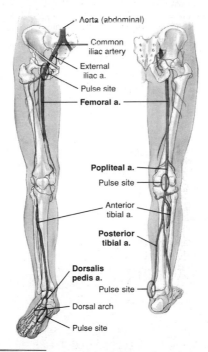

► Figure 14–1   Arteries and arterial pulse sites in the leg

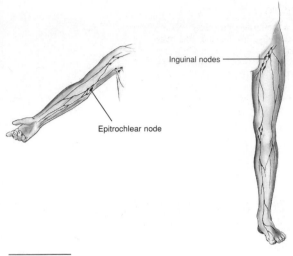

Inguinal nodes

Epitrochlear node

► Figure 14-2   Lymphatics in the extremities

The *lymphatics* form a completely separate vessel system, which retrieves excess fluid from the tissue spaces and returns it to the blood stream. The lymphatic system also forms a major part of the immune system that defends the body against disease.

Cervical lymph nodes drain the head and neck and are described in Chapter 6. Axillary lymph nodes drain the breast and upper arm and are described in Chapter 10.

The *epitrochlear* lymph node is in the antecubital fossa and drains the hand and lower arm (Fig. 14-2). The *inguinal* nodes in the groin drain most of the lymph of the lower extremity, the external genitalia, and the anterior abdominal wall.

SUBJECTIVE DATA

Leg pain or cramps.

Skin changes on arms or legs

Swelling in legs

Lymph node enlargement (swollen glands)

OBJECTIVE DATA

Equipment Needed

Occasionally need: Paper tape measure
Tourniquet or BP cuff
Stethoscope

Preparation

During a complete physical examination, examine the arms at the very beginning when you are checking the vital signs—the person is sitting. Examine the legs directly after the abdominal examination while the person is still supine. Then stand the person up to evaluate the leg veins.

METHOD OF EXAMINATION

NORMAL RANGE OF FINDINGS	ABNORMAL FINDINGS

THE ARMS

Inspect and Palpate the Arms

Note color of skin and nailbeds, temperature, texture, and turgor of skin, and the presence of any lesions, edema, or clubbing as described in Chapter 5.

The two arms should be symmetric in size.

Edema of upper extremities is uncommon but does occur when lymphatic drainage is obstructed, as seen following some type of breast surgery (see Table 18–2, p. 658 in Jarvis: *Physical Examination and Health Assessment*).

Note the presence of any scars on hands and arms. Many occur normally with usual childhood abrasions or with occupations involving hand tools.

Needle tracks in antecubital fossae occur with intravenous drug use; linear scars in wrists may signify past self-inflicted injury.

Palpate both radial pulses, noting rate, rhythm, elasticity of vessel wall, and equal force. Grade the force (amplitude) on a four-point scale:

4+, bounding
3+, increased
2+, **normal**
1+, weak
0, absent

Weak thready pulse, full bounding pulse, dropped beats, irregular pulse (see Table 14–1, pp. 155–156).

Palpate the brachial pulses—their force should be equal bilaterally. Check the epitrochlear lymph node in the depression above and behind the medial condyle of the humerus.

An enlarged epitrochlear node occurs with infection of the hand or forearm.

NORMAL RANGE OF FINDINGS	ABNORMAL FINDINGS

THE LEGS
Inspect and Palpate the Legs

Inspect both legs together, noting skin color, hair distribution, venous pattern, size (swelling or atrophy), and any skin lesions or ulcers.

Pallor with vasoconstriction; erythema with vasodilatation; cyanosis.

Ulcers occur both with chronic arterial insufficiency and with chronic venous insufficiency (see Table 18–4, p. 659 in Jarvis: *Physical Examination and Health Assessment*).

Hair normally covers the legs. Even if leg hair is shaved, you will still note hair on the dorsa of the toes.

Malnutrition: thin, shiny atrophic skin, thick-ridged nails, loss of hair, ulcers, gangrene.

Malnutrition, pallor, and coolness occur with arterial insufficiency.

The venous pattern is normally flat and barely visible. Note obvious varicosities although these are best assessed while standing.

Both legs should be symmetric in size without swelling or atrophy. If the lower legs appear asymmetric, measure the calf circumference with a nonstretchable tape measure. Measure at the widest point, in exactly the same place, the same number of centimeters down from the patella or other landmark. Record your findings in centimeters.

Diffuse bilateral edema occurs with systemic illnesses.

Unilateral swelling indicates a local acute problem.

Using the dorsa of your hands, palpate for temperature from the feet up along the legs, comparing symmetric spots. The skin should be warm and equal bilaterally. Bilateral cool feet may be due to environmental factors such as cool room temperature, apprehension, and cigarette smoking. If there is any increase in temperature up the leg, note if it is gradual or abrupt.

A unilateral cool foot or leg occurs with arterial deficit.

Palpate the inguinal lymph nodes. It is not unusual to find palpable nodes that are small (1 cm or less), movable, and nontender.

Enlarged nodes, tender or fixed in area.

Palpate these peripheral arteries in both legs: femoral, popliteal, dorsalis pedis, and posterior tibial. Grade the force on the four-point scale.

NORMAL RANGE OF FINDINGS	ABNORMAL FINDINGS

Femoral Pulse. Locate the femoral arteries just below the inguinal ligament halfway between the pubis and anterior-superior iliac spines (see Fig. 14–1). To help expose the femoral area, particularly in obese people, ask the person to bend his or her knees to the side in a froglike position. Press firmly and then slowly release, noting the pulse tap under your fingertips. Should this pulse be weak or diminished, auscultate the site for a bruit.

A bruit occurs with turbulent blood flow, indicating arterial occlusion.

Popliteal pulse. This is a more diffuse pulse and can be difficult to localize. Bend the knees up a little, anchor your thumbs on the knee, and curl fingers around into the fossa. Push forward against the bone. Use a light touch and search the area. It is often just lateral to the medial tendon. Often, a normal popliteal pulse is impossible to palpate.

Posterior Tibial Pulse. Curve your fingers around the medial malleolus (Fig. 14–3). You will feel the tapping right behind it in the groove between the malleolus and the Achilles tendon.

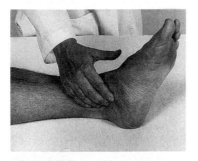

▶ Figure 14–3   Posterior tibial pulse

Dorsalis Pedis Pulse. This requires a very light touch. It is normally just lateral to and parallel with the extensor tendon of the big toe (Fig. 14–4).

NORMAL RANGE OF FINDINGS	ABNORMAL FINDINGS

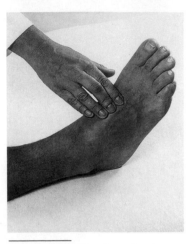

▶ Figure 14–4   Dorsalis pedis pulse

Check for pretibial edema. Firmly depress the skin over the tibia or the medial malleolus for 5 seconds and release. Your finger should normally leave no indentation, although a pit is commonly seen if the person has been standing all day or during pregnancy. If pitting edema is present, grade it on this scale:

1+ mild, slight depression
to
4+ severe, deep depression.

This scale is subjective.

Ask the person to stand in order to assess the venous system. Note any visible, dilated, and tortuous veins.

ADDITIONAL TECHNIQUES

The Doppler Ultrasonic Flowmeter. Use this device to detect a weak peripheral pulse, to monitor blood pressure in infants or children, or to measure a low blood pressure or blood pressure in a lower extremity (Fig. 14–5). The Doppler flowmeter magnifies pulsatile sounds from the heart and blood vessels. Place a drop of coupling gel on the end of

Bilateral, dependent, pitting edema occurs with congestive heart failure and hepatic cirrhosis.

Unilateral edema occurs with occlusion of a deep vein and unilaterally or bilaterally with lymphatic obstruction. With these factors, it is "brawny" or nonpitting and feels hard to the touch.

Varicosities occur in the saphenous veins (see Table 18–4, pp. 659–660 in Jarvis: *Physical Examination and Health Assessment*).

NORMAL RANGE OF FINDINGS	ABNORMAL FINDINGS

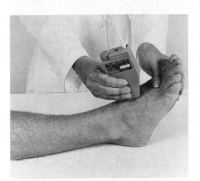

▶ Figure 14–5   Using the Doppler to locate a pulse

the hand-held transducer. Place the transducer over a pulse site, tilted at a 45-degree angle. Locate the pulse site by the swishing whooshing sound.

DEVELOPMENTAL CONSIDERATIONS

Infants and Children

Transient acrocyanosis (i.e. symmetric cyanosis of the hands and wrists, feet and ankles) and skin mottling may occur at birth. Pulse force should be normal and symmetric. Pulse force should also be the same in the upper and lower extremities.

Weak pulses occur with vasoconstriction or diminished cardiac output.

Full bounding pulses occur with patent ductus arteriosus due to the large left-to-right shunt.

Diminished or absent femoral pulses, while upper extremity pulses are normal, suggests coarctation of aorta.

Palpable lymph nodes occur often in normal infants and children. They are small, firm (shotty), mobile, and nontender. They may be the sequelae of past infection, e.g., inguinal nodes from a diaper rash or cervical nodes from a respiratory infection. Vaccinations can also produce local lymphadenopathy. Note characteristics of any palpable nodes and whether they are local or generalized.

Enlarged, warm, tender nodes indicate current infection. Look for source.

NORMAL RANGE OF FINDINGS	ABNORMAL FINDINGS

The Pregnant Female

Expect diffuse, bilateral, pitting edema in the lower extremities, especially at the end of the day and into the third trimester. Varicose veins in the legs are also common in the third trimester.

The Aging Adult

The dorsalis pedis and posterior tibial pulses may become more difficult to find. Trophic changes associated with arterial insufficiency (thin shiny skin, thick-ridged nails, loss of hair on lower legs) also occur normally with aging.

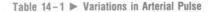

A B N O R M A L   F I N D I N G S

Table 14-1 ▶ Variations in Arterial Pulse

Description	Associated With
Weak "Thready" Pulse—1+. Hard to palpate, need to search for it, may fade in and out, easily obliterated by pressure.	Decreased cardiac output; peripheral arterial disease; aortic valve stenosis.
Full Bounding Pulse—3+ or 4+. Easily palpable, pounds under your fingertips.	Hyperkinetic states (exercise, anxiety, fever), anemia, hyperthyroidism.
Water-Hammer (Corrigan's Pulse—4+. Greater than normal force, then collapses suddenly.	Aortic valve regurgitation; patient ductus arteriosus.
Pulsus bigeminus. Rhythm is coupled, every other beat comes early, or normal beat followed by premature beat. Force of premature beat is decreased due to shortened cardiac filling time.	Conduction disturbance, e.g., premature ventricular contraction, premature atrial contraction.
Pulsus Alternans. Rhythm is regular but force varies with alternating beats of large and small amplitude.	Left-sided congestive heart failure.
Pulsus Paradoxus. Beats have weaker amplitude with inspiration, stronger with expiration. Best determined during blood pressure measurement; reading decreases (>10 mmHg) during inspiration and increases with expiration.	Cardiac tamponade; constrictive pericarditis.

Inspiration   Expiration   Inspiration

Table 14-1 ► **Variations in Arterial Pulse** *Continued*

Description	Associated With

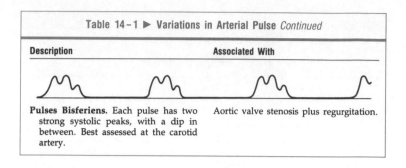

Pulses Bisferiens. Each pulse has two strong systolic peaks, with a dip in between. Best assessed at the carotid artery.

Aortic valve stenosis plus regurgitation.

☑ **SUMMARY CHECKLIST**

1 ► Inspect arms for color, size, any lesions
2 ► Palpate pulses: radial, brachial
3 ► Check epitrochlear node
4 ► Inspect legs for color, size, any lesions, trophic skin changes

5 ► Palpate temperature of feet and legs
6 ► Palpate inguinal nodes
7 ► Palpate pulses: femoral, popliteal, posterior tibial, dorsalis pedis

Nursing Diagnoses Commonly Associated with Peripheral Vascular System

Altered tissue perfusion: peripheral

Activity intolerance

Altered tissue integrity

Body image disturbance

Fatigue

Pain

Sleep pattern disturbance

Sensory perceptual alteration: tactile

Sexual dysfunction

15 Musculoskeletal System

The musculoskeletal system consists of the bones, joints, and muscles.

The joint (or articulation) is the place of union of two or more bones. Joints are the functional units of the musculoskeletal system because they permit the mobility needed for activities of daily living.

Synovial joints are freely movable because they have bones that are separated from each other and which are enclosed in a joint cavity (Fig. 15–1). This cavity is filled with a lubricant, or synovial fluid.

In synovial joints, a layer of resilient *cartilage* covers the surface of opposing bones. The cartilage cushions the bones and gives a smooth surface to facilitate movement. The joint is surrounded by a fibrous capsule and is supported by ligaments. *Ligaments* are fibrous bands running

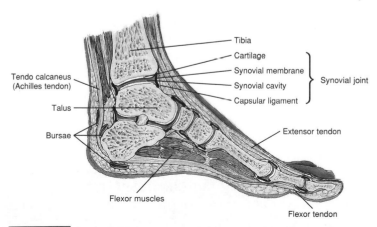

▶ Figure 15–1   Components of a synovial joint

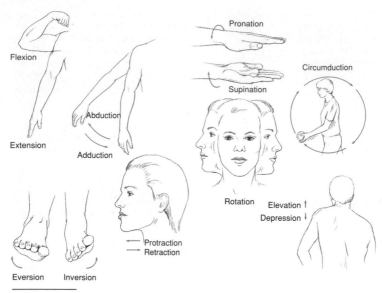

▶ Figure 15-2   Movements of skeletal muscles

directly from one bone to another that strengthen the joint and help prevent movement in undesirable directions. A *bursa* is an enclosed sac filled with viscous synovial fluid, much like a joint. Bursae are located in areas of potential friction (e.g., subacromial bursa of the shoulder, prepatellar bursa of the knee) and help muscles and tendons glide smoothly over bone.

The skeletal muscle is attached to bone by a *tendon*—a strong fibrous cord. Skeletal muscles produce the following movements (Fig. 15-2):

1. flexion—bending a limb at a joint
2. extension—straightening a limb at a joint
3. abduction—moving a limb away from the midline of the body
4. adduction—moving a limb toward the midline of the body
5. pronation—turning the forearm so the palm is down
6. supination—turning the forearm so the palm is up
7. circumduction—moving the arm in a circle around the shoulder
8. inversion—moving the sole of the foot inward at the ankle
9. eversion—moving the sole of the foot outward at the ankle
10. rotation—moving the head around a central axis
11. protraction—moving a body part forward and parallel to the ground
12. retraction—moving a body part backward and parallel to the ground
13. elevation—raising a body part
14. depression—lowering a body part

TRANSCULTURAL CONSIDERATIONS

The long bones of blacks are significantly longer, narrower, and denser than those of whites (Farrally and Moore,

1975). Bone density measured by race and sex reveal that black males have the densest bones, thus accounting for the relatively low incidence of osteoporosis in this population. Bone density in the Chinese, Japanese, and Eskimos is below that of white Americans (Garn, 1964).

S U B J E C T I V E   D A T A

Joints
  pain
  stiffness
  swelling, heat
  limitation of movement

Muscles
  pain (cramps)
  weakness

Bones
  pain
  deformity
  trauma (fractures, sprains, dislocations)

Functional assessment (ADL)
  any self-care deficit in: bathing, toileting, dressing, grooming, eating, communicating, mobility. Use of mobility aids

Self-care behaviors
  occupational hazards
    heavy lifting
    repetitive motion to joints
  nature of exercise program
  recent weight gain

O B J E C T I V E   D A T A

Equipment Needed

  Tape measure
  Goniometer to measure joint angles
  Skin-marking pen

Preparation

The purpose of the musculoskeletal examination is to assess function for activities of daily living (ADL), as well as to screen for any abnormalities.

A *screening* musculoskeletal examination suffices for most people:

• Inspection and palpation of joints integrated with each body region
• Observation of ROM as person proceeds through motions necessary for an examination
• Age-specific screening measures, e.g., scoliosis screening for adolescents

A *complete* musculoskeletal examination, as described in this chapter, is appropriate for persons with articular disease, a history of musculoskeletal symptoms, or any problems with ADL.

METHOD OF EXAMINATION

NORMAL RANGE OF FINDINGS	ABNORMAL FINDINGS

ORDER OF THE EXAMINATION

Use the following order for each specific joint.

Inspection

Compare corresponding paired joints. Inspect for symmetry of structure and function as well as normal parameters for that joint.

Note the *size* and *contour* of the joint. Inspect the skin and tissues over the joints for *color, swelling,* and *masses* or *deformity.*

Presence of swelling is significant and signals joint irritation.

Palpation

Palpate each joint, including its skin for temperature, its muscles, bony articulations, and area of joint capsule. Notice any heat, tenderness, swelling, or masses. Joints are normally not tender to palpation.

Heat, tenderness and swelling signal inflammation.
  Mass.

Range of Motion (ROM)

Ask for *active* range of motion while stabilizing the body area proximal to that being moved. Familiarize yourself with the type of each joint and its normal range of motion so you can recognize limitations. If you see a limitation, gently attempt *passive* motion. Anchor the joint with one hand while your other hand slowly moves it to its limit. The normal ranges of active and passive motion should be the same.

If any limitation or increase in ROM occurs, use a goniometer to precisely measure the angles (Fig. 15–3). First extend the joint to neutral or 0 degrees. Center the 0 point of the goniometer on the joint. Keep the fixed arm of the goniometer on the 0 line and use the movable arm to measure; then flex the joint and measure through the goniometer to

NORMAL RANGE OF FINDINGS   ABNORMAL FINDINGS

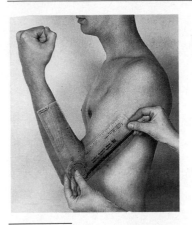

▶ Figure 15–3   Measuring joint motion
with a goniometer

determine the angle of greatest flexion.

Joint motion normally causes no
tenderness, pain, or crepitation.
Crepitation is an audible and palpable crunching or grating that accompanies movement. Do not confuse
crepitation with the normal, discrete
"crack" heard as a tendon or ligament slips over bone during motion,
such as when you do a knee bend.

Crepitation occurs when the articular surfaces in the joints are
roughened, as with rheumatoid
arthritis.

Muscle Testing

Test the strength of the prime
mover muscle groups for each joint.
Repeat the motions you elicited for
active ROM. Now ask the person to
flex and hold as you apply opposing
force. Muscle strength should be
equal bilaterally and should fully re-
sist your opposing force. (Note:
Muscle status and joint status are
interdependent and should be inter-
preted together. Chapter 16 dis-
cusses the examination of muscles
for size and development, tone, and
presence of tenderness).

There is a wide variability of
strength among people. You may
wish to use a grading system from
no voluntary movement to full
strength, as shown in Table 15–1
on p. 175.

NORMAL RANGE OF FINDINGS	ABNORMAL FINDINGS

CERVICAL SPINE

Inspect the alignment of head and neck. The spine should be straight and the head erect. Palpate the spinous processes and the sternomastoid, trapezius, and paravertebral muscles. They should feel firm, with no muscle spasm or tenderness.

Ask the person to follow these motions:*

INSTRUCTIONS TO PERSON	MOTION AND EXPECTED RANGE
• Touch chin to chest	Flexion of 45 degrees
• Lift the chin toward the ceiling	Hyperextension of 55 degrees
• Touch each ear toward the corresponding shoulder. Do not lift up the shoulder	Lateral bending of 40 degrees
• Turn the chin toward each shoulder	Rotation of 70 degrees

* DO NOT ATTEMPT IF YOU SUSPECT NECK TRAUMA

Repeat the motions while applying opposing force. The person can normally maintain flexion against your full resistance. This also tests integrity of cranial nerve XI.

UPPER EXTREMITY

Shoulder

Inspect and compare both shoulders posteriorly and anteriorly. Check the size and contour of the joint and compare shoulders for equality of bony landmarks. There is normally no redness, muscular atrophy, deformity, or swelling.

While standing in front of the person, palpate both shoulders, noting any muscular spasm or atrophy, swelling, heat, or tenderness.

Test ROM by asking the person to perform four motions. Cup one hand over the shoulder during ROM to note any crepitation; normally there is none.

ABNORMAL FINDINGS column:

Head tilted to one side.
Asymmetry of muscles.
Tenderness.
Hard muscles with muscle spasm.

Limited ROM.
Pain with movement.

The person cannot hold flexion.

Redness.
Inequality of bony landmarks.
Atrophy, shows as lack of fullness (see Table 19–4, pp. 716–717 in Jarvis: *Physical Examination and Health Assessment*).

Swelling.
Hard muscles with muscle spasm.
Tenderness or pain.

NORMAL RANGE OF FINDINGS		ABNORMAL FINDINGS

INSTRUCTIONS TO PERSON	MOTION AND EXPECTED RANGE	
1. With arms at sides and elbows extended, move both arms forward and up in wide vertical arcs. Then move them back.	Forward flexion of 180 degrees. Hyperextension up to 50 degrees.	Limited ROM. Asymmetry. Pain with motion. Crepitus with motion.
2. Rotate arms internally behind back, place back of hands as high as possible toward the scapulae.	Internal rotation of 90 degrees.	
3. With arms at sides and elbows extended, raise both arms in wide arcs in the coronal plane. Touch palms together above head.	Abduction of 180 degrees. Adduction of 50 degrees.	
4. Touch both hands behind the head, with elbows flexed and rotated posteriorly.	External rotation of 90 degrees.	

Test the strength of the shoulder muscles by asking the person to shrug the shoulders, flex forward and up, and abduct against your resistance. The shoulder shrug also tests the integrity of cranial nerve XII.

Elbow

Inspect the size and contour of the elbow in both flexed and extended positions. Look for any deformity, redness, or swelling.

Test ROM by asking the person to:

Swelling and redness (see Table 19–5, p. 718 in Jarvis: *Physical Examination and Health Assessment*).

INSTRUCTIONS TO PERSON	MOTION AND EXPECTED RANGE
• Bend and straighten the elbow.	Flexion of 150–160 degrees, extension at 0. Some normal people lack 5–10 degrees of full extension, and others have 5–10 degrees of hyperextension.
• Hold the hand midway, then touch front and back sides of hand to table.	Movement of 90 degrees in pronation and supination.

NORMAL RANGE OF FINDINGS

ABNORMAL FINDINGS

While testing muscle strength, stabilize the person's arm with one hand (Fig. 15–4). Have the person flex the elbow against your resistance, applied just proximal to the wrist. Then ask the person to extend the elbow against your resistance.

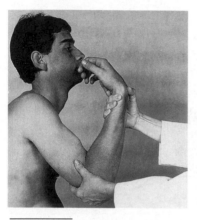

▶ Figure 15–4 Stabilize the joint while testing muscle strength

Wrist and Hand

Inspect the hands and wrists on the dorsal and palmar sides, noting position, contour, and shape. The normal functional position of the hand shows the wrist in slight extension. This way the fingers can flex efficiently, and the thumb can oppose them for grip and manipulation. The fingers lie straight in the same axis as the forearm. There is normally no swelling or redness, deformity, or nodules.

The skin looks smooth, with knuckle wrinkles present and no swelling or lesions. Muscles are full, with the palm showing a rounded mound proximal to the thumb (the *thenar eminence*), and a smaller rounded mound proximal to the little finger.

Subluxation of wrist.
Ulnar deviation; fingers list to ulnar side.
Ankylosing; wrist in extreme flexion.
Dupuytren's contracture; flexion contracture of finger(s).
Swan neck or boutonniere deformity in fingers.
Hard nodules on fingers (see Table 19–6, pp. 719–721 in Jarvis: *Physical Examination and Health Assessment*).

Atrophy of the thenar eminence.

NORMAL RANGE OF FINDINGS	ABNORMAL FINDINGS

Palpate each joint in the wrist and hands. Facing the person, support the hand with your fingers under it. Use gentle but firm pressure. Normally, the joint surfaces feel smooth, with no swelling, bogginess, nodules, or tenderness.

Ganglion in wrist.
Synovial swelling on dorsum.
Generalized swelling.
Tenderness.

Test ROM by using this procedure:

INSTRUCTIONS TO PERSON	MOTION AND EXPECTED RANGE	
• Bend the hand up at the wrist.	Hyperextension of 70 degrees	Loss of ROM here is the most common and the most significant type of functional loss of the wrist.
• Bend hand down at the wrist.	Palmar flexion of 90 degrees.	Limited motion.
• Bend the fingers up and down at meta-carpophalangeal joints	Flexion of 90 degrees. Hyperextension of 30 degrees.	
• With palms flat on table, turn them outward and in.	Ulnar deviation of 50–60 degrees, and radial deviation of 20 degrees.	Pain on movement.
• Spread fingers apart; make a fist.	Abduction of 20 degrees; fist tight. The responses should be equal bilaterally.	
• Touch the thumb to each finger and to the base of little finger.	The person is able to perform, and the responses are equal bilaterally.	

LOWER EXTREMITY

Hip

Wait to inspect the hip joint together with the spine a bit later in the examination as the person stands. At that time, note symmetric levels of iliac crests, gluteal folds, and equally sized buttocks. A smooth, even gait reflects equal leg lengths and functional hip motion.

Help the person into a supine position, and palpate the hip joints. The joints should feel stable and symmetric, with no tenderness or crepitance.

Pain with palpation.
Crepitation.

Assess ROM by asking the person to:

NORMAL RANGE OF FINDINGS	ABNORMAL FINDINGS

INSTRUCTIONS TO PERSON	MOTION AND EXPECTED RANGE	
• Raise each leg with knee extended	Hip flexion of 90 degrees	Limited motion. Pain with motion. Flexion flattens the lumbar spine; if this reveals a flexion deformity in the opposite hip, it is abnormal.
• Bend each knee up to the chest while keeping the other leg straight.	Hip flexion of 120 degrees. The opposite thigh should remain on the table.	
• Flex knee and hip to 90 degrees. Stabilize by holding the thigh with one hand and the ankle with the other hand. Swing the foot outward. Swing the foot inward. (Foot and thigh move in opposing directions.)	Internal rotation of 40 degrees. External rotation of 45 degrees.	Limited internal rotation of hip is an early and reliable sign of hip disease.
• Swing leg laterally, then medially, with knee straight. Stabilize pelvis by pushing down on the opposite anterior-superior iliac spine.	Abduction of 40–45 degrees, adduction of 20–30 degrees.	Limitation of abduction of the hip while supine is the most common motion dysfunction found in hip disease.
• When standing (later in examination), swing straight leg back behind body. Stabilize pelvis to eliminate exaggerated lumbar lordosis.	Hyperextension of 15 degrees when stabilized.	

Knee

The skin normally looks smooth, with even coloring and free of lesions.

Inspect lower leg alignment. The lower leg should extend in the same axis as the thigh.

Inspect the knee's shape and contour. Normally, there are distinct concavities, or hollows, on either side of the patella. Check them for any sign of fullness or swelling. Note other locations, such as the prepatellar bursa and the suprapatellar pouch, for any abnormal swelling.

Check the quadriceps muscle in the anterior thigh for any atrophy. Since it is the prime mover of knee extension, this muscle is important for joint stability during weight-bearing.

Calluses.
Shiny and atrophic skin.
Inflammation.
Lesions, e.g., psoriasis.
Angulation deformity.
Flexion contracture.

Hollows disappear, then may bulge with synovial thickening or effusion (see Table 19–7, pp. 722–723 in Jarvis: *Physical Examination and Health Assessment*).

Atrophy occurs with disuse or chronic disorders. It first appears in the medial part of the muscle, although it is difficult to note because the vastis medialis is relatively small.

NORMAL RANGE OF FINDINGS	ABNORMAL FINDINGS

Check ROM by asking the person to:

INSTRUCTIONS TO PERSON	MOTION AND EXPECTED RANGE	
• Bend each knee	Flexion of 130–150 degrees	Limited in ROM.
• Extend each knee.	A straight line of 0 degrees, in some persons; a hyperextension of 15 degrees in others.	Contracture. Pain with motion.
• Check knee ROM during ambulation.		Limp.\ \ Sudden locking—the person is unable to extend the knee fully. This usually occurs with a painful and audible "pop" or "click."\ \ Sudden buckling, or "giving way," occurs with ligament injury, which causes weakness and instability.

Check muscle strength by asking the person to maintain knee flexion while you oppose by trying to pull the leg forward. Muscle extension is demonstrated by the person's success in rising from a seated position in a low chair or by rising from a squat without using the hands for support.

Ankle and Foot

Inspect and compare both feet, noting position of feet and toes, contour of joints, and skin characteristics. The foot should align with the long axis of the lower leg.

The toes point straight forward and lie flat. The ankles (malleoli) are smooth, bony prominences. The skin is normally smooth, with even coloring and no lesions. Note the locations of any calluses or bursal reactions because they reveal areas of abnormal friction. Examining well-worn shoes helps assess areas of wear and accommodation.

Test ROM by asking the person to:

Hallux valgus and bunion.
Hammer toes.
Claw toes.
Swelling or inflammation.
Calluses.
Ulcers.
(See Table 19–8, pp. 724–725 in Jarvis: *Physical Examination and Health Assessment.*)

INSTRUCTIONS TO PERSON	MOTION AND EXPECTED RANGE	
• Point toes toward the floor.	Plantar flexion of 45 degrees.	Limited ROM.
• Point toes toward your nose.	Dorsiflexion of 20 degrees.	Pain with motion.
• Turn soles of feet out, then in. (Stabilize the ankle with one hand, hold heel	Eversion of 20 degrees.\ Inversion of 30 degrees.	

NORMAL RANGE OF FINDINGS	ABNORMAL FINDINGS

with the other to test the subtalar joint.)
• Flex and straighten toes.

Assess muscle strength by asking the person to maintain dorsiflexion and plantar flexion against your resistance.

Unable to hold flexion.

SPINE

The person should be standing, draped in a gown open at the back. Place yourself far enough back so that you can see the entire back. Note if the spine is straight by following an imaginary vertical line from the head through the spinous processes and down through the gluteal cleft, and by noting equal horizontal positions for the shoulders, scapulae, iliac crests, and gluteal folds, and equal spaces between arm and lateral thorax on the two sides (Fig. 15–5A). The person's knees and feet should be aligned with the trunk and should be pointing forward.

From the side, note the normal convex thoracic curve and concave lumbar curve (see Fig. 15–5B). An

A difference in shoulder elevation and in level of scapulae and iliac crests occurs with scoliosis (see Table 15–2 on pp. 175–176).

Lateral tilting and forward bending occur with a herniated nucleus pulposus.

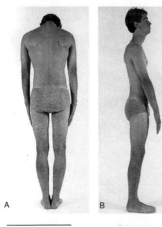

A   B

▶ Figure 15–5 (A) Straight spine
(B) Normal curvature seen from side

NORMAL RANGE OF FINDINGS	ABNORMAL FINDINGS

enhanced thoracic curve, or kyphosis, is common in aging people. A
pronounced lumbar curve, or lordosis, is common in obese people (see
Table 15–2 on pp. 175–176).

Check ROM of the spine by asking the person to bend forward and
touch the toes. Look for flexion of
75–90 degrees and smoothness and
symmetry of movement. Note that
the concave lumbar curve should
disappear with this motion, and the
back should have a single, convex,
C-shaped curve.

Stabilize the pelvis with your
hands. Check ROM by asking the
person to:

INSTRUCTIONS TO PERSON	MOTION AND EXPECTED RANGE	
• Bend sideways.	Lateral bending of 35 degrees.	Limited ROM.
• Bend backward.	Hyperextension of 30 degrees.	Pain with motion.
• Twist shoulders to one side, then the other.	Rotation of 30 degrees, bilaterally.	

DEVELOPMENTAL CONSIDERATIONS

Infants

Lift up the infant and examine the
back. Note the normal, single, C-
curve of the newborn's spine (Fig.
15–6). By 2 months of age, the

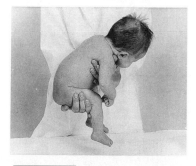

▶ Figure 15–6   Normal spinal curvature in newborn

NORMAL RANGE OF FINDINGS	ABNORMAL FINDINGS

infant can lift the head while prone. This builds the concave cervical spinal curve and indicates normal forearm strength.

Observe ROM through spontaneous movement of extremities.

Test muscle strength by lifting up the infant, with your hands under the baby's axillae. A baby with normal muscle strength wedges securely between your hands.

A baby who starts to "slip" between your hands shows weakness of the shoulder muscles.

Preschool and School-Aged Children

Once the infant learns to crawl and then to walk, the waking hours show perpetual motion. This is convenient for your musculoskeletal assessment—you can observe the muscles and joints during spontaneous play before a table-top examination. Most young children enjoy showing off their physical accomplishments. For specific motions coax the toddler, "Show me how you can walk to Mom," ". . . climb the step stool." Ask the preschooler to hop on one foot or to jump.

While the child is standing, note the posture. From behind, you should note a "plumb line" from the back of the head, along the spine, to the middle of the sacrum. Shoulders are level within 1 cm and scapulae are symmetrical. From the side, lordosis is common throughout childhood, appearing more pronounced in children with a protuberant abdomen.

Lordosis is marked with muscular dystrophy and rickets.

Check the child's gait while walking away from and returning to you. Let the child wear socks, because a cold tile floor will distort the usual gait.

Limp; usually caused by trauma, fatigue, or hip disease.

From 1 to 2 years of age, expect a broad-based gait, with arms out for balance. Weight-bearing falls on the inside of the foot. From 3 years of age, the base narrows and the arms are closer to the sides. Inspect the shoes for spots of greatest wear to aid your judgment of the gait. Normally, the shoes wear more on the

NORMAL RANGE OF FINDINGS	ABNORMAL FINDINGS

outside of the heel and the inside of the toe.

Adolescents

Proceed with the musculoskeletal examination you provide for the adult, except pay special note to spinal posture. Kyphosis is common during adolescence because of chronic poor posture.

Screen for *scoliosis* starting at age 12 (Fig. 15-7). Seat yourself behind the standing child, and ask the child to bend forward to touch the toes. Expect a straight vertical spine while standing and also while bending forward. Posterior ribs should be symmetric, with equal elevation of shoulders, scapulae, and iliac crests. You may wish to mark each spinous process with a felt marker when the adolescent bends forward. The line-up of ink dots when she or he stands up highlights even a subtle curve.

Scoliosis is exhibited as ribs hump up on one side as child bends forward and with unequal landmark elevation (see Table 15-2).

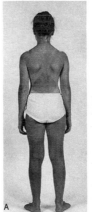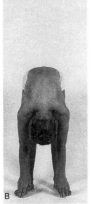

▶ Figure 15-7   Scoliosis screening

Be aware of the risk of sports-related injuries with the adolescent, because sports participation and competition reach a height with this age group.

NORMAL RANGE OF FINDINGS	ABNORMAL FINDINGS

The Pregnant Female

Proceed through the examination described in the adult section. Expected postural changes in pregnancy include progressive lordosis and, toward the third trimester, anterior cervical flexion, kyphosis, and slumped shoulders. When the pregnancy is at term, the protuberant abdomen and the relaxed mobility in the joints create the characteristic "waddling" gait.

The Aging Adult

Postural changes include a decrease in height, more apparent in the eighth and ninth decades (Fig. 15–8). "Lengthening of the arm-trunk

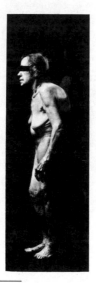

► Figure 15–8

axis" describes this shortening of the trunk with comparatively long extremities. Kyphosis is common, with a backward head tilt to compensate. This creates the outline of a figure 3 when you view this older adult

NORMAL RANGE OF FINDINGS   ABNORMAL FINDINGS

from the left side. Slight flexion of
hips and knees is also common.

Contour changes include a decrease of fat in the body periphery
and fat deposition over the abdomen and hips. The bony prominences become more marked.

For most older adults, ROM testing proceeds as described earlier.
ROM and muscle strength are much
the same as with the younger adult,
provided there are no musculoskeletal illnesses or arthritic changes.

Functional Assessment

For those with advanced aging
changes, arthritic changes, or musculoskeletal disability, perform a
functional assessment for ADL. This
applies the range of motion and
muscle strength assessments to the
accomplishment of specific activities.
You need to determine adequate
and safe performance of functions
essential for independent home life.

INSTRUCTIONS TO PERSON	COMMON ADAPTATION FOR AGING CHANGES*
1 ▶ Walk (with shoes on)	Shuffling pattern; swaying; arms out to help balance; broader base of support; person may watch feet.
2 ▶ Climb up stairs	Person holds hand rail; may haul body up with it; may lead with favored (stronger) leg.
3 ▶ Walk down stairs	Holds hand rail, sometimes with both hands. If the person is weak, he or she may descend sideways lowering the weaker leg first. If the person is unsteady, he or she may watch feet.
4 ▶ Pick up object from floor	Person often bends at waist instead of bending knees; holds furniture to support while bending and straightening.

NORMAL RANGE OF FINDINGS   ABNORMAL FINDINGS

5 ▶ Rise up from sitting in chair	Person uses arms to push off chair arms, upper trunk leans forward before body straightens, feet planted wide in broad base of support.
6 ▶ Rise up from lying in bed.	May roll to one side, push with arms to lift up torso, grab bedside table to increase leverage.

* Data from Bowers AC, Thompson MJ:
Clinical Manual of Health Assessment, 3rd ed.
St. Louis, CV Mosby, 1988.

A B N O R M A L   F I N D I N G S

Table 15-1 ▶ Grading Muscle Strength

GRADE	DESCRIPTION	PERCENT NORMAL	ASSESSMENT
5	Full ROM against gravity, full resistance	100	Normal
4	Full ROM against gravity, some resistance	75	Good
3	Full ROM with gravity	50	Fair
2	Full ROM with gravity eliminated (passive motion)	25	Poor
1	Slight contraction	10	Trace
0	No contraction	0	Zero

Table 15-2 ▶ Curvatures of the Spine

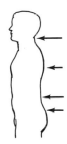

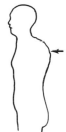

NORMAL SPINAL CURVATURE

The vertebral column has four curves (a double S shape). The cervical and lumbar curves are concave (inward), and the thoracic and sacrococcygeal curves are convex. The balanced or compensatory nature of these curves, together with the resilient intervertebral discs, allows the spine to absorb a great deal of shock.

KYPHOSIS

An exaggerated posterior curvature of the thoracic spine (humpback), associated with aging. Compensation may occur by hyperextension of head to maintain level of vision.

Table 15–2 ▶ Curvatures of the Spine *Continued*

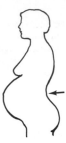

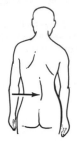

LORDOSIS

The normal lumbar concavity is further accentuated, associated with pregnancy, obesity, or kyphosis.

LIST

The spine tilts to one side, away from the affected side, usually associated with pressure on the local spinal nerve root from a herniated disc.

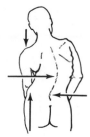

SCOLIOSIS

A lateral S-shaped curvature of the thoracic and lumbar spine, usually with involved vertebrae rotation. Note rib hump on forward flexion. When standing, note unequal shoulder and scapular height, obvious curvature, unequal elbow level, unequal hip levels, and rib interspaces flared on convex side. More prevalent in adolescence, especially in girls.

✓ SUMMARY CHECKLIST

For each joint to be examined:
1 ▶ Inspection
   Size and contour of joint
   Skin color and characteristics
2 ▶ Palpation of joint area
   Skin
   Muscles
   Bony articulations
   Joint capsule

3 ▶ ROM
   Active
   Passive (if there is limitation in active ROM)
   Measure with goniometer (if there is abnormality in ROM)
4 ▶ Muscle testing

Nursing Diagnoses Commonly Associated with the Musculoskeletal Disorders

Activity intolerance

Altered growth and development

Body image disturbance

Chronic pain

Diversional activity deficit

Impaired home maintenance management

Impaired skin integrity

Impaired physical mobility

Pain

Potential for disuse syndrome

Potential for trauma

Self-care deficit

Sleep pattern disturbance

The nervous system can be divided into two parts—central and peripheral. The *central nervous system* (CNS) includes the brain and spinal cord. The *peripheral nervous system* includes the 12 pairs of cranial nerves, the 31 pairs of spinal nerves, and all their branches. The peripheral nervous system carries messages *to* the CNS from sensory receptors and *from* the CNS out to muscles and glands.

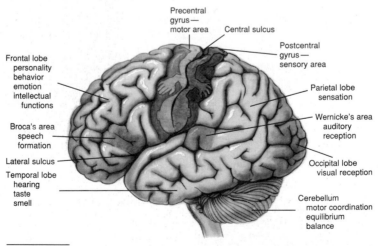

Precentral gyrus—motor area

Central sulcus

Postcentral gyrus—sensory area

Frontal lobe
personality
behavior
emotion
intellectual
functions

Parietal lobe
sensation

Wernicke's area
auditory
reception

Broca's area
speech
formation

Lateral sulcus

Temporal lobe
hearing
taste
smell

Occipital lobe
visual reception

Cerebellum
motor coordination
equilibrium
balance

▶ Figure 16-1   The lobes of the cerebral cortex and their specific functions

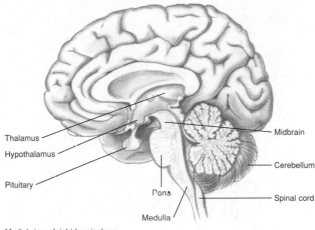

Thalamus

Hypothalamus

Pituitary

Pons

Medulla

Midbrain

Cerebellum

Spinal cord

Medial view of right hemisphere

▶ Figure 16-2   Components of the CNS

THE CENTRAL NERVOUS SYSTEM (CNS)

Cerebral Cortex

The cerebral cortex is the cerebrum's outer layer of nerve cell bodies, also called gray matter. The cerebral cortex is the center for human's highest functions, governing thought, memory, reasoning, sensation, and voluntary movement (Fig. 16-1).

Each half of the cerebrum is a *hemisphere*. Each hemisphere is divided into four *lobes:* frontal, parietal, temporal, and occipital.

The lobes have certain areas that mediate certain functions as labelled in Fig. 16-1. Damage to these specific cortical areas produces a corresponding loss of function: motor deficit, paralysis, loss of sensation, or impaired ability to understand and process language.

Components of the CNS

In addition to the cerebral cortex, the CNS has other vital components (Fig. 16-2).

The *thalamus* is the main relay station for incoming sensory pathways.

The *hypothalamus* controls temperature, sleep, emotions, autonomic activity, and the pituitary gland.

The *cerebellum* is concerned with motor coordination, equilibrium, and muscle tone.

The *midbrain* and *pons* contain motor neurons and motor and sensory tracts. The *medulla* contains fiber tracts, and vital autonomic centers for respiration, heart, and gastrointestinal function.

The *spinal cord* is the main highway for ascending and descending fiber tracts that connect the brain to the spinal nerves, and it mediates reflexes.

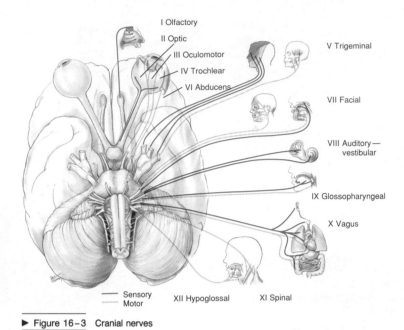

I Olfactory
II Optic
III Oculomotor
IV Trochlear
VI Abducens
V Trigeminal
VII Facial
VIII Auditory—vestibular
IX Glossopharyngeal
X Vagus
Sensory
Motor
XII Hypoglossal   XI Spinal

▶ Figure 16–3   Cranial nerves

THE PERIPHERAL NERVOUS SYSTEM

Cranial Nerves

Cranial nerves enter and exit the brain rather than the spinal cord (Fig. 16–3). The 12 pairs of cranial nerves supply primarily the head and neck, with the exception of the vagus nerve which travels to the heart, respiratory muscles, stomach, and gallbladder.

Spinal Nerves

The 31 pairs of spinal nerves arise from the length of the spinal cord and supply the rest of the body (Fig. 16–4). They are named for the region of the spine from which they exit: 8 cervical, 12 thoracic, 5 lumbar, 5 sacral, and 1 coccygeal. They

are "mixed" nerves because they contain both sensory and motor fibers.

Reflex Arc

In the most simple reflex, the sensory afferent fibers carry the message from the receptor and travel through the dorsal root into the spinal cord (Fig. 16–5). They synapse in the cord with the motor neuron in the anterior horn. Motor efferent fibers leave via the ventral root and travel to the muscle.

The deep tendon or stretch reflex has five components:

1. An intact sensory nerve (afferent)
2. A functional synapse in the cord
3. An intact motor nerve fiber (efferent)
4. The neuromuscular junction
5. A competent muscle.

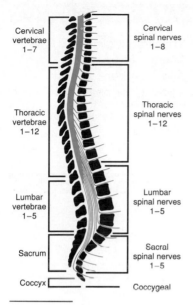

Cervical vertebrae 1–7

Thoracic vertebrae 1–12

Lumbar vertebrae 1–5

Sacrum

Coccyx

Cervical spinal nerves 1–8

Thoracic spinal nerves 1–12

Lumbar spinal nerves 1–5

Sacral spinal nerves 1–5

Coccygeal

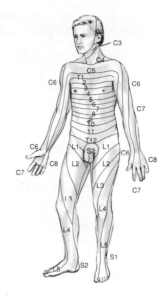

▶ Figure 16–4   Spinal nerves

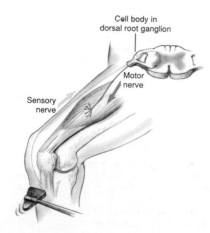

Cell body in dorsal root ganglion

Motor nerve

Sensory nerve

▶ Figure 16–5   Reflex arc

S U B J E C T I V E   D A T A

Headache (unusually frequent or severe)

Head injury

Dizziness (feeling lightheaded or faint)/ vertigo (feeling a rotational spinning)

Seizures

Tremors

Weakness or incoordination

Numbness or tingling

Difficulty swallowing

Difficulty speaking

Significant neurologic past history (stroke, spinal cord injury, meningitis or encephalitis, congenital defect, alcoholism)

O B J E C T I V E   D A T A

Equipment Needed

Penlight

Tongue blade

Sterile needle

Cotton ball

Tuning fork (128 Hz)

Percussion hammer

Preparation

Perform a *screening* neurologic examination (items identified in following sections) on seemingly well persons who have no significant subjective findings from the history.

Perform a *neurologic recheck* examination on persons with demonstrated neurologic deficits who require periodic assessments (e.g., hospitalized persons or those in extended care), using the exam sequence beginning on page 196.

METHOD OF EXAMINATION

NORMAL FINDINGS	ABNORMAL FINDINGS
MENTAL STATUS Assess level of consciousness (see Chapter 2 and exam sequence on p. 9).	

NORMAL RANGE OF FINDINGS	ABNORMAL FINDINGS

CRANIAL NERVES
Test Selected Cranial Nerves

Cranial Nerve II — Optic Nerve

Test visual acuity and test visual fields by confrontation (Chapter 7). When indicated, use the ophthalmoscope to examine the ocular fundus (see Chapter 7).

Visual field loss (see Table 11–2, p. 348 in Jarvis: *Physical Examination and Health Assessment*).

Papilledema with increased intracranial pressure; optic atrophy (see Table 11–11, p. 358 in Jarvis: *Physical Examination and Health Assessment*).

Cranial Nerves III, IV, and VI — Oculomotor, Trochlear, and Abducens Nerves

Palpebral fissures are usually equal in width or nearly so.

Ptosis (drooping) with myasthenia gravis, dysfunction of cranial nerve III, or Horner's syndrome (see Table 7–2 on p. 67).

Check pupils for size, regularity, equality, light reaction, and accommodation (see Chapter 7). The pupils are normally equal, round, react to light promptly and react to accommodation, or PERRLA.

Unequal size, constricted pupils, dilated pupils, or no response to light. See Table 7–3 on p. 68.

Assess extraocular movements by the cardinal positions of gaze (see Chapter 7).

Nystagmus is a back-and-forth oscillation of the eyes. End-point nystagmus, a few beats of horizontal nystagmus at extreme lateral gaze, occurs normally. Assess any other nystagmus carefully.

Deviated gaze or limited movement.

Cranial Nerve V — Trigeminal Nerve

Motor Function. Palpate the temporal and masseter muscles as the person clenches the teeth. Muscles should feel equally strong on both sides. Try to separate the jaws by pushing down on the chin; normally you cannot.

Decreased strength on one or both sides.

Pain with clenching of teeth.

Sensory Function. With the person's eyes closed, test light touch sensation

NORMAL RANGE OF FINDINGS	ABNORMAL FINDINGS

by touching a cotton wisp to these designated areas on person's face: forehead, cheeks, and chin. Ask the person to say "Now," whenever the touch is felt.

Decreased or unequal sensation.

Cranial Nerve VII—Facial Nerve

Motor Function. Note mobility and facial symmetry as the person responds to these requests: smile, frown, close eyes tightly (against your attempt to open them), lift eyebrows, show teeth, and puff cheeks.

Muscle weakness is shown by loss of the nasolabial fold, drooping of one side of the face, lower eyelid sagging, and escape of air from only one puffed cheek when both are pressed in.

THE MOTOR SYSTEM

Inspect and Palpate the Motor System

Muscles

Size. Muscle groups should be within the normal size limits for age and should be symmetric bilaterally. When muscles in the extremities appear asymmetric, measure each in centimeters and record the difference. A difference of 1 cm or less is not significant. Note that it is difficult to assess muscle mass in very obese people.

Atrophy—abnormally small muscle with a wasted appearance; occurs with disuse, injury, lower motor neuron disease, and muscle disease.

Hypertrophy—increased size and strength; occurs with isometric exercise.

Strength. (See Chapter 15, Musculoskeletal System) Test homologous muscles simultaneously.

Cerebellar Function

Gait. Observe as the person walks 10 to 20 feet, turns, and returns to the starting point. Normally, the gait is smooth, rhythmic, and effortless; the opposing arm swing is coordinated; the turns are smooth. The step length is about 15 inches from heel to heel.

Stiff, immobile posture.
Staggering or reeling.
Wide base of support.
Lack of arm swing or rigid arms.
Unequal rhythm of steps.
Slapping of foot.
Scraping of toe of shoe.
Ataxia—uncoordinated or unsteady gait (see Table 16–1 on pp. 200, 201, and 202).
Crooked line of walk.
Widens base to maintain balance.

Ask the person to walk a straight line in a heel-to-toe fashion (tandem walking) (Fig. 16–6). This decreases

NORMAL RANGE OF FINDINGS	ABNORMAL FINDINGS

the base of support and will accentuate any problem with coordination. Normally, the person can walk straight and stay balanced.

Staggering, reeling, loss of balance.

An ataxia that did not appear with regular gait may now appear.

Romberg's Test. Ask the person to stand up with feet together and arms at the sides. Once in a stable position, ask the person to close the eyes and hold the position (Fig. 16–7). Wait about 20 seconds. Normally, a person can maintain posture and balance, although there may be slight swaying. (Stand close to catch the person in case he or she falls).

Sways; falls; widens base of feet to avoid falling.

Positive Romberg's sign is loss of balance increased by closing of the eyes; occurs with cerebellar ataxia (multiple sclerosis, alcohol intoxication), loss of proprioception, and loss of vestibular function.

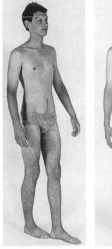 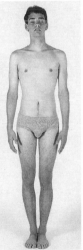

▶ Figure 16–6   ▶ Figure 16–7

Walk heel-to-toe   Romberg's test

Ask the person to perform a shallow knee bend or to hop in place, first on one leg, then the other. This demonstrates normal position sense, muscle strength, and cerebellar function. Note that some individuals cannot hop due to aging or obesity.

NORMAL RANGE OF FINDINGS	ABNORMAL FINDINGS

THE SENSORY SYSTEM

Assess the Sensory System

Make sure the person is alert, cooperative, comfortable, and has an adequate attention span; otherwise, you may get misleading and invalid results. Testing of the sensory system can be fatiguing. You may need to repeat the examination later or break it into parts when the person tires.

Routine screening procedures include testing superficial pain, light touch, vibration in a few distal locations, and stereognosis.

The person's eyes should be closed during each test. Take time to explain what will be happening and exactly how you expect the person to respond.

Superficial Pain

Using a sterile needle, lightly apply the sharp point and the dull hub to the person's body in a random, unpredictable order (Fig. 16–8). Ask the person to say "sharp" or "dull," depending on the sensation felt. (Note that the sharp edge is used to test for pain; the dull edge is used as a general test of the person's responses.) Alternatively break a tongue blade lengthwise, forming a sharp point at the fractured end, and using the dull spot at the rounded end.*

Let at least 2 seconds elapse between each stimulus to avoid *summation*. With summation, frequent consecutive stimuli are perceived as one strong stimulus.

Hypalgesia—decreased pain sensation.

Analgesia—absent pain sensation.

Hyperalgesia—increased pain sensation.

(See Table 20–9, pp. 791–792 in Jarvis: *Physical Examination and Health Assessment.*)

---

*To prevent any possible contagion, do not reuse a needle or sharp tool on another person. Dispose of needles or any sharp tools in a special impenetrable container.

NORMAL RANGE OF FINDINGS   ABNORMAL FINDINGS

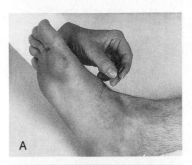

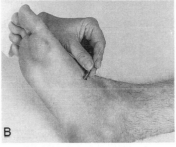

▶ Figure 16-8   Test superficial pain

Light Touch

Apply a wisp of cotton to the skin. Stretch a cotton ball to make a long end and brush it over the skin in a random order of sites and at irregular intervals. Ask the person to say "now" or "yes" when touch is felt. Compare symmetric points.

Hypesthesia—decreased touch sensation.
Anesthesia—absent touch sensation.
Hyperesthesia—increased touch sensation.

Vibration

Strike a low-pitch tuning fork on the heel of your hand and hold the base on a bony surface of the fingers and great toe. Ask the person to indicate when the vibration starts and stops. The normal response is vibration or buzzing sensation on these distal areas. If no vibrations are felt, move proximally and test ulnar processes, ankles, patellae, and iliac crests. Compare the right side to the left. If you find a deficit, note whether it is gradual or abrupt.

Unable to feel vibration. States vibration stops when fork is still vibrating.
Loss of vibration sense occurs with peripheral neuropathy, e.g., diabetes and alcoholism. This is often the first sensation lost.

NORMAL RANGE OF FINDINGS

ABNORMAL FINDINGS

Stereognosis

Test the person's ability to recognize objects by feeling their forms, sizes, and weights. With the eyes closed, place a familiar object (paper clip, key, coin, cotton ball, or pencil) in the person's hand and ask the person to identify it (Fig. 16–9). A person will normally explore it with the fingers and correctly name it. Test a different object in each hand; testing the left hand assesses right parietal lobe functioning.

Astereognosis—unable to identify object correctly. Occurs in sensory cortex lesions.

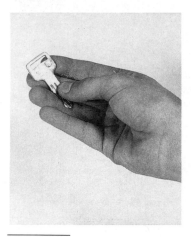

▶ Figure 16–9   Stereognosis

REFLEXES

Test the Reflexes

Stretch, or Deep Tendon Reflexes (DTRs)

For an adequate response, the limb should be relaxed and the muscle partially stretched. Stimulate the reflex by directing a short snappy blow of the reflex hammer onto the muscle's insertion tendon. Strike a brief, well-aimed blow and bounce up promptly; do not let the hammer

NORMAL RANGE OF FINDINGS   ABNORMAL FINDINGS

rest on the tendon. Use the pointed end of the reflex hammer when aiming at a smaller target (such as your thumb) on the tendon site; use the flat end when the target is wider or to diffuse the impact and prevent pain.

Use just enough force to get a response. Compare right and left sides—the responses should be equal. The reflex response is graded on a 4-point scale:

4+ very brisk, hyperactive with clonus, indicative of disease

3+ brisker than average, may indicate disease

2+ average, normal

1+ diminished, low normal

0   no response

Clonus is a set of short, jerking contractions of the same muscle.

Hyperreflexia is the exaggerated reflex seen when the monosynaptic reflex arc is released from the influence of higher cortical levels. This occurs with upper motor neuron lesions, e.g., a cerebrovascular accident.

Hyporeflexia, which is the absence of a reflex, is a lower motor neuron problem. It occurs with interruption of sensory afferents or destruction of motor efferents and anterior horn cells, e.g., spinal cord injury.

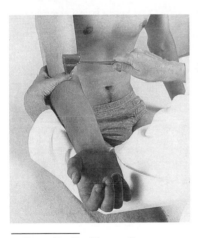

▶ Figure 16–10   Biceps reflex

Biceps Reflex (C-5 to C-6). Support the person's forearm on yours; this position relaxes as well as partially flexes the person's arm. Place your thumb on the biceps tendon and strike a blow on your thumb. You can feel as well as see the normal response which is flexion of the forearm (Fig 16–10).

NORMAL RANGE OF FINDINGS	ABNORMAL FINDINGS

Triceps Reflex (C-7 to C-8). Tell the person to let the arm "just go dead" as you suspend it by holding the upper arm. Strike the triceps tendon directly just above the elbow (Fig. 16–11). The normal response is extension of the forearm. Alternately, hold the person's wrist across the chest to flex the arm at the elbow, and tap the tendon.

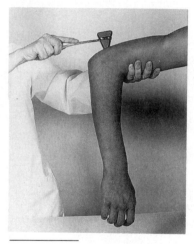

▶ Figure 16–11   Triceps reflex

Patellar Reflex ("Knee Jerk") (L-2 to L-4). Let the lower legs dangle freely to flex the knee and stretch the tendons. Strike the tendon directly just below the patella (Fig. 16–12). Extension of the lower leg is the expected response. You also will palpate the contraction of the quadriceps.

Achilles Reflex ("Ankle Jerk") (L-5 to S-2). Position the person with the knee flexed and the hip externally rotated. Hold the foot in dorsiflexion

NORMAL RANGE OF FINDINGS	ABNORMAL FINDINGS

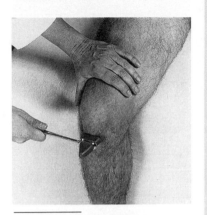

▶ Figure 16–12   Patellar reflex

and strike the Achilles tendon directly (Fig. 16–13). Feel the normal response as the foot plantar flexes against your hand.

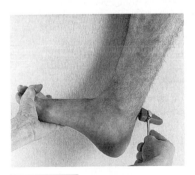

▶ Figure 16–13   Achilles reflex

Plantar Reflex (L-4 to S-2). With the end of the reflex hammer, draw a light stroke up the lateral side of the sole of the foot and across the ball of the foot, like an upside-down "J" (Fig. 16–14). The normal response is plantar flexion of the toes and sometimes of the entire foot.

Except in infancy, the abnormal response is dorsiflexion of the big toe and fanning of all toes, which is a *positive Babinski's* sign. This occurs with upper motor neuron disease of the pyramidal tract.

NORMAL RANGE OF FINDINGS	ABNORMAL FINDINGS

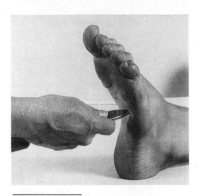

▶ Figure 16–14   Plantar reflex

DEVELOPMENTAL CONSIDERATIONS

Infants (Birth to 12 Months)

Assessment includes noting that milestones you normally would expect for each month have indeed been achieved and that the early, more primitive reflexes are eliminated from the baby's repertory when they are supposed to.

Observe spontaneous motor activity for smoothness and symmetry. Smoothness of movement suggests proper cerebellar function, as does the coordination involved in sucking and swallowing. To screen gross and fine motor coordination, use the Denver-II developmental screening test with its age-specific developmental milestones (see pp. 42–45 in Jarvis: *Physical Examination and Health Assessment*).

Check the muscle tone necessary for head control. With the baby supine and holding the wrists, pull to a sit and note head control. The newborn will hold the head in almost the same plane as the body, and the head will balance briefly when the baby reaches a sitting position, then flop forward. (Even a

Failure to attain a skill by expected time.

Persistence of reflex behavior beyond the normal time.

Delay in motor activity occurs with brain damage, mental retardation, peripheral neuromuscular damage, prolonged illness, and parental neglect.

Because development progresses in a cephalocaudal direction, head lag is an early sign of brain damage.

NORMAL RANGE OF FINDINGS	ABNORMAL FINDINGS

premature infant shows some head flexion). At 4 months of age, the head stays in line with the body and does not flop.

Reflexes have a predictable timetable of appearance and departure. For the screening examination, check the rooting, grasp, Babinski's, tonic neck, and Moro reflexes.

Rooting Reflex. Brush the infant's cheek near the mouth. The infant normally turns the head toward that side and opens the mouth. The reflex appears at birth and disappears within 3 to 4 months.

Palmar Grasp. Offer your finger and note tight grasp of all the baby's fingers. Sucking enhances grasp. You can often pull baby to a sit from grasp. The reflex is present at birth, is strongest at 1 to 2 months, and disappears at 3 to 4 months.

Babinski's Reflex. Stroke your finger up the lateral edge and across the ball of the infant's foot. Note fanning of toes (positive Babinski's reflex—Figure 16–15). The reflex is present at birth and disappears (changes to the adult response) by 24 months of age (variable).

After 6 months of age, any baby with failure to hold head in midline when sitting should be referred.

The reflex is absent with brain damage and with local muscle or nerve injury.

Persistence of the reflex after 4 months of age occurs with frontal lobe lesion.

Positive Babinski's reflex after 2 or 2½ years of age occurs with pyramidal tract disease.

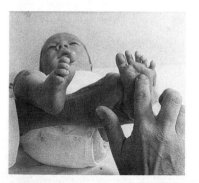

▶ Figure 16–15   Babinski's reflex

NORMAL RANGE OF FINDINGS	ABNORMAL FINDINGS

Tonic Neck Reflex. With the baby supine, relaxed, or sleeping, turn the head to one side with the chin over shoulder. Note ipsilateral extension of the arm and leg and flexion of the opposite arm and leg; this is the "fencing" position. If you turn the infant's head to the opposite side, positions will reverse (Fig. 16–6). The reflex appears by 2 to 3 months, decreases at 3 to 4 months, and disappears by 4 to 6 months.

Persistence later in infancy occurs with brain damage.

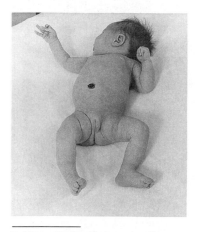

▶ Figure 16–16   Tonic nerve reflex

Moro Reflex. Startle the infant by jarring the crib, making a loud noise, or supporting the head and back in a semisitting position and quickly lower the infant to 30 degrees. The baby looks as if he or she is "grasping a tree" (Barness, 1981); that is, there is symmetric abduction and extension of the arms and legs, fanning fingers, and curling the index finger and thumb to C-position. The infant then brings in both arms and legs (Fig. 16–17). The reflex is present at birth and disappears at 1 to 4 months.

Absence of the Moro reflex in the newborn or persistence after 5 months of age indicates severe CNS injury.

Absence of movement in one arm occurs with fracture of the humerus or clavicle, and brachial nerve palsy.

Absence in one leg occurs with a lower spinal cord problem or a dislocated hip.

A hyperactive Moro reflex occurs with tetany or CNS infection.

NORMAL RANGE OF FINDINGS   ABNORMAL FINDINGS

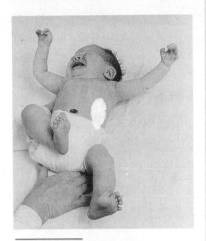

▶ Figure 16–17   Moro reflex

The Aging Adult

Use the same examination as used with the younger adult. Be aware that some aging adults show a slower response to your requests, especially to those calling for coordination of movements.

Any decrease in muscle bulk is most apparent in the hand, as seen by guttering between the metacarpals. These dorsal hand muscles often look wasted, even with no apparent arthopathy. The grip strength remains relatively good.

Senile tremor occasionally occur. These benign tremors include an intention tremor of the hands, head nodding (as if saying yes or no), and tongue protrusion. There is no associated rigidity.

The gait may be slower, more deliberate, and may deviate slightly from a midline path than that in the younger person.

After 65 years of age, loss of the sensation of vibration at the ankle malleolus is common and is usually accompanied by loss of the ankle jerk. Tactile sensation may be impaired. The aging person may need

Hand muscle atrophy is worsened with disuse and degenerative arthropathy.

Distinguish senile tremors from tremors of parkinsonism. The latter includes rigidity, and slowness and weakness of voluntary movement.

Absence of a rhythmic, reciprocal gait pattern is seen in parkinsonism and hemiparesis (see Table 16–1 on p. 200).

Note any difference in sensation between right and left sides, which may indicate a neurologic deficit.

NORMAL RANGE OF FINDINGS	ABNORMAL FINDINGS

stronger stimuli for light touch and especially pain.

The DTRs are less brisk. Those in the upper extremities are usually present, but the ankle jerks are commonly lost. Knee jerks may be lost, but this occurs less often.

The plantar reflex may be absent or difficult to interpret. Often you will not see a definite normal flexor response; however, you should still consider a definite extensor response to be abnormal.

NEUROLOGIC RECHECK

Some hospitalized persons have head trauma or a neurologic deficit due to a systemic disease process. These people must be monitored closely for any improvement or deterioration in neurologic status and for any indication of increasing intracranial pressure. Signs of increasing intracranial pressure signal impending cerebral disaster and death and require early and prompt intervention.

Use an abbreviation of the neurologic examination in the following sequence:
1. Level of consciousness
2. Motor function
3. Pupillary response
4. Vital signs

Level of Consciousness. A *change* in the level of consciousness is the single most important factor in this examination. It is the earliest and most sensitive index of change in neurologic status. Note the ease of *arousal* and the state of awareness, or *orientation.* Assess orientation by asking questions about:
person—own name, occupation, names of workers around person, their occupation
place—where person is, nature of building, city, state
time—day of week, month, year

Vary the questions during repeat assessments so that the person is not

A change in consciousness may be subtle. Note any decreasing level of consciousness, disorientation, memory loss, uncooperative behavior, or even complacency in a previously combative person.

NORMAL RANGE OF FINDINGS

ABNORMAL FINDINGS

merely memorizing answers. Note the quality and content of the verbal response; articulation, fluency, manner of thinking, and any deficit in language comprehension or production (see Chapter 2, pp. 9–11).

A person is fully alert when his or her eyes open at your approach or spontaneously; when he or she is oriented to person, place, and time; and when he or she is able to follow verbal commands appropriately.

If the person is not fully alert, increase the amount of stimulus used in this order:

name called
light touch on person's arm
vigorous shake of shoulder
pain applied (pinch nailbed, pinch trapezius muscle, rub your knuckles on the person's sternum)

Record the stimulus used as well as the person's response to it.

Motor Function. Check the voluntary movement of each extremity by giving the person specific commands. (This procedure also tests level of consciousness by noting the person's ability to follow commands).

Ask the person to lift the eyebrows, frown, bare teeth. Note symmetric facial movements and bilateral nasolabial folds (cranial nerve VII).

Check upper arm strength by checking hand grasps. Ask the person to squeeze your fingers. Offer your two fingers, one on top of the other, so that a strong hand grasp does not hurt your knuckles.

Check lower extremities by asking the person to do straight leg raises. Ask the person to lift one leg at a time straight up off the bed. Full strength allows the leg to be lifted 90 degrees. If multiple trauma, pain, or equipment preclude this motion, ask the person to push one foot at a time against your hand's resistance,

Review Table 2–2, Levels of Consciousness, Chapter 2, p. 10.

NORMAL RANGE OF FINDINGS	ABNORMAL FINDINGS

"like putting your foot on the gas pedal of your car."

For the person with decreased level of consciousness, note if movement occurs spontaneously, and as a result of noxious stimuli, such as pain or suctioning. An attempt to push away your hand after such stimuli is called *localizing* and is characterized as purposeful movement.

Any normal posturing, decorticate rigidity, or decerebrate rigidity indicates diffuse brain injury (see Table 20–10, p. 793 in Jarvis: *Physical Examination and Health Assessment*).

Pupillary Response. Note the size, shape, and symmetry of both pupils. Shine a light into each pupil and note the direct and consensual light reflex. Both pupils should constrict briskly. (Allow for the effects of any medication that could affect pupil size and reactivity). When recording, pupil size is best expressed in millimeters. Tape a millimeter scale onto a tongue blade and hold it next to the person's eyes for the most accurate measurement (Fig. 16–18).

In a brain-injured person, a sudden, unilateral, dilated and nonreactive pupil is ominous. Cranial nerve III runs parallel to the brain stem. When increasing intracranial pressure pushes the brain stem down (uncal herniation), it puts pressure on cranial nerve III, causing pupil dilation.

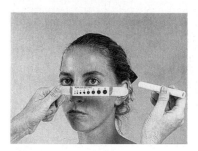

▶ Figure 16–18   Measure pupil size in millimeters

Vital Signs. Measure the temperature, pulse, respiration, and blood pressure as often as the person's condition warrants. Although they are vital to the overall assessment of the critically ill person, pulse and blood pressure are notoriously unreliable parameters of CNS deficit. Any changes are late consequences of rising intracranial pressure.

Signs of increasing intracranial pressure, the *Cushing reflex:* Blood pressure—sudden elevation with widening pulse pressure; Pulse—decreased rate, slow and bounding.

NORMAL RANGE OF FINDINGS   ABNORMAL FINDINGS

The Glasgow Coma Scale (GCS).
The GCS is an objective assessment
that defines the level of consciousness by giving it a numerical value
(Fig. 16–19).

The scale is divided into three
areas: eye opening, verbal response,
and motor response. Each area is
rated separately, and a number is
given for the person's best response.
The three numbers are added; the
total score reflects the brain's functional level. A fully alert, normal
person has a score of 15, whereas a
score of 7 or less reflects coma. Serial assessments can be plotted on a
graph to illustrate visually whether
the person is stable, improving, or
deteriorating.

GLASGOW COMA SCALE		
BEST EYE OPENING RESPONSE (Record "C" if eyes closed by swelling)	Spontaneously	4
	To speech	3
	To pain	2
	No response	1
BEST MOTOR RESPONSE to painful stimuli (Record best upper limb response)	Obeys verbal command	6
	Localizes pain	5
	Flexion — withdrawal	4
	Flexion — abnormal*	3
	Extension — abnormal**	2
	No response	1
BEST VERBAL RESPONSE (Record "E" if endotracheal tube in place. "T" if tracheostomy tube in place)	Oriented × 3	5
	Conversation — confused	4
	Speech — inappropriate	3
	Sounds — incomprehensible	2
	No response	1
	* abnormal flexion — decorticate rigidity ** abnormal extension — decerebrate rigidity	

▶ Figure 16–19

ABNORMAL FINDINGS

Table 16-1 ▶ Abnormal Gaits

TYPE	CHARACTERISTIC APPEARANCE	POSSIBLE CAUSE
Spastic hemiparesis 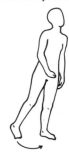	Arm is immobile against the body, with flexion of the shoulder, elbow, wrist, fingers, and adduction of shoulder. The leg is stiff and extended, and circumducts with each step (drags toe in a semicircle).	Upper motor neuron lesion of the corticospinal tract, e.g., cerebrovascular accident, trauma.
Cerebellar ataxia 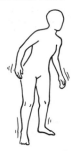	Staggering, wide-based gait; difficulty with turns; uncoordinated movement with positive Romberg's sign.	Alcohol or barbiturate effect on cerebellum; cerebellar tumor; multiple sclerosis.
Parkinsonian (festinating) 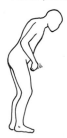	Posture is stooped; trunk is pitched forward; elbows, hips, and knees are flexed. Steps are short and shuffling. Hesitation to begin walking, and difficulty stopping suddenly. The person holds the body rigid. Walks and turns body as one fixed unit. Difficulty with any change in direction.	Parkinsonism.

| Table 16–1 ► Abnormal Gaits *Continued* | | |

TYPE	CHARACTERISTIC APPEARANCE	POSSIBLE CAUSE
Scissors	Knees cross or are in contact, like holding an orange between the thighs. The person uses short steps, and walking requires effort.	Paraparesis of legs, multiple sclerosis
Steppage or footdrop	Slapping quality — looks as if walking up stairs and finds no stair there. Lifts knee and foot high and slaps it down hard and flat to compensate for footdrop.	Weakness of peroneal and anterior tibial muscles; due to lower motor neuron lesion at the spinal cord, e.g., poliomyelitis, Charcot-Marie-Tooth disease.
Waddling	Weak hip muscles — when the person takes a step, the opposite hip drops, which allows compensatory lateral movement of pelvis. Often, the person also has marked lumbar lordosis and a protruding abdomen.	Hip girdle muscle weakness due to muscular dystrophy, dislocation of hips.

	CHARACTERISTIC	
TYPE	APPEARANCE	POSSIBLE CAUSE
Short leg	Leg length discrepancy >2.5 cm (1 inch). Vertical telescoping of affected side, which dips as the person walks. Appearance of gait varies depending on amount of accompanying muscle dysfunction.	Congenital dislocated hip; acquired shortening due to disease, trauma.

Table 16–1 ▶ Abnormal Gaits *Continued*

☑ SUMMARY CHECKLIST

Neurologic Screening Examination

1 ▶ Mental Status (level of consciousness)
2 ▶ Cranial Nerves
   II Optic
   III, IV, VI—Extraocular muscle
   V Jaw muscles and facial sensation
   VII Facial mobility
3 ▶ Motor function
   Gait and balance
   Knee flexion—hop or shallow knee bend

4 ▶ Sensory function
   Superficial pain and light touch—arms and legs
   Vibration—arms and legs
   Stereognosis
5 ▶ Reflexes
   Biceps
   Triceps
   Patellar
   Achilles
   Plantar

Nursing Diagnoses Commonly Associated with Nervous System—Neurologic Disorders

Activity intolerance

Body image disturbance

Diversional activity deficit

Dysreflexia

Fear

Home maintenance management

Impaired physical mobility

Impaired swallowing

Impaired verbal communication

Ineffective thermoregulation

Ineffective individual coping

Potential for trauma

Reflex incontinence

Sensory perceptual alteration: kinesthetic

Sensory perceptual alteration: tactile, visual

Skin integrity, potential impaired

Total incontinence

Unilateral neglect

Urinary elimination, altered patterns of

17 Male Genitalia

The male genitalia include the penis and scrotum externally, and the testis, epididymis and vas deferens internally (Fig. 17–1). The accessory glandular structures (the prostate, seminal vesicles) are discussed in Chapter 19.

The *urethra* transverses the penis, and its meatus forms a slit at the glans tip.

The *scrotum* is a loose sac, which is a continuation of the abdominal wall. In each scrotal half is a *testis,* which produces sperm. The testis has a solid oval shape and is about 4 to 5 cm long by 3 cm wide in the adult.

The testis is capped by the *epididymis,* which is a markedly coiled duct system. The epididymis is con-

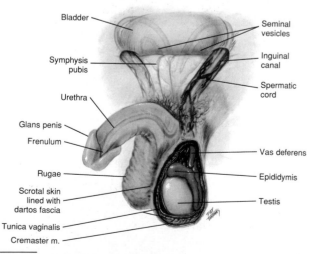

Bladder
Seminal vesicles
Symphysis pubis
Inguinal canal
Spermatic cord
Urethra
Glans penis
Frenulum
Vas deferens
Rugae
Epididymis
Scrotal skin lined with dartos fascia
Testis
Tunica vaginalis
Cremaster m.

▶ Figure 17–1 The male genital structures

tinuous with the *vas deferens,* which approximates with other vessels to form the *spermatic cord.* The spermatic cord runs through the inguinal canal into the abdomen.

Puberty begins sometime between ages 9½ to 13½. The first sign is enlargement of the testes. Next, pubic hair appears; then penis size increases. The stages of development are documented in Tanner's sexual maturity ratings (SMR) (Table 17–1 on p. 210).

The complete change in male genitalia development from preadolescent to adult takes around 3 years, although the normal range is 2 to 5 years.

SUBJECTIVE DATA

Frequency, urgency, and nocturia

Dysuria (pain or burning with urination)

Hesitancy and straining

Urine color (cloudy or hematuria)

Past genitourinary history (kidney disease, kidney stones, flank pain, urinary tract infections, prostate trouble)

Penis — pain, lesion, discharge

Scrotum — pain, lumps

Self-care behaviors — perform testicular self-examination

Sexual activity and contraceptive use

Sexually transmitted disease (STD) contact

OBJECTIVE DATA

Equipment Needed

Gloves — Wear gloves during every male genitalia examination

Occasionally: glass slide for urethral specimen

Flashlight

Preparation

Position the male standing with undershorts down and appropriate draping. The examiner should be sitting. Alternatively, the male may be supine for the first part of the examination and stand to check for a hernia.

METHOD OF EXAMINATION

NORMAL RANGE OF FINDINGS	ABNORMAL FINDINGS
PENIS	
Inspect and Palpate the Penis	
The skin normally looks wrinkled, hairless, and without lesions.	Generalized swelling. Inflammation.

NORMAL RANGE OF FINDINGS	ABNORMAL FINDINGS
	Lesions: nodules, solitary ulcer (chancre), grouped vesicles or superficial ulcers, wartlike papules (see Table 21–2 in Jarvis: *Physical Examination and Health Assessment,* p. 821).
The glans looks smooth and without lesions. Ask the uncircumcised male to retract the foreskin or you retract it. It should move easily. After inspection, slide the foreskin back to the original position. The urethral meatus is positioned just about centrally on the glans.	Phimosis—unable to retract the foreskin. Paraphimosis—unable to return foreskin to original position. Hypospadias—ventral location of meatus. Epispadias—dorsal location of meatus (see Table 21–3 in Jarvis: *Physical Examination and Health Assessment,* p. 822). Stricture—narrowed opening.
Compress the glans anteroposteriorly between your thumb and forefinger. The edge of the meatus should appear pink, smooth, and without discharge.	Edges that are red, everted, edematous, along with purulent discharge, suggest urethritis (see Table 21–4, p. 823 in Jarvis: *Physical Examination and Health Assessment*).
Palpate—the penis normally feels smooth, semifirm, and nontender.	Nodule. Induration. Tenderness.

SCROTUM

Inspect and Palpate the Scrotum

Scrotal size varies with ambient room temperature. Asymmetry is normal, with the left scrotal half lower than the right. Lift the sac to inspect the posterior surface. Normally, there are no scrotal lesions except for the commonly found sebaceous cysts. These are yellowish, 1-cm nodules that are firm, nontender and often multiple.	Scrotal swelling (edema) may be taut and pitting. This occurs with congestive heart failure, renal failure, or local inflammation. Lesions. Inflammation.
Palpate each scrotal half between your thumb and first two fingers. Testes normally feel oval, firm and rubbery, smooth and equal bilaterally, and are freely movable and slightly tender to moderate pressure. Each epididymis normally feels discrete, softer than the testis, smooth, and nontender.	Absent testis—may be a temporary migration or true cryptorchidism (see Table 21–5 in Jarvis: *Physical Examination and Health Assessment,* pp. 824–826). Atrophied testes—small and soft. Fixed testes. Nodules on testes or epididymides. Marked tenderness.

NORMAL RANGE OF FINDINGS	ABNORMAL FINDINGS

Between your thumb and forefinger, palpate each spermatic cord along its length, from the epididymis up to the external inguinal ring. It should feel smooth and nontender.

Normally, there are no other scrotal contents. If you do find a mass, note:

- Is there any tenderness?
- Is the mass distal or proximal to testis?
- Can you place your fingers over it?
- Does it reduce when person lies down?
- Can you auscultate bowel sounds over it?

Thickened.

Soft, swollen, and tortuous— see the discussion of varicocele, Table 21–5 in Jarvis: *Physical Examination and Health Assessment,* pp. 824–826.

Abnormalities in the scrotum: hernia, tumor, orchitis, epididymitis, hydrocele, spermatocele, varicocele (see Table 21–5 in Jarvis: *Physical Examination and Health Assessment,* pp. 824–826).

HERNIA

Inspect and Palpate for Hernia

Inspect the inguinal region for a bulge as the person stands and as he strains down. Normally there is none.

Bulge at external inguinal ring, or femoral canal. (A hernia may be present but easily reduced and appears only intermittently with an increase in intra-abdominal pressure.)

Palpate the inguinal canal (Fig. 17–2). Ask the male to shift his weight onto the unexamined leg. Place your index finger low on the scrotal half. Palpate up the length of

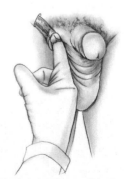

▶ Figure 17–2   Palpate for inguinal hernia

NORMAL RANGE OF FINDINGS	ABNORMAL FINDINGS

the spermatic cord, invaginating the scrotal skin as you go, to the external inguinal ring. The inguinal ring feels like a triangular, slitlike opening, and it may or may not admit your finger. If it will will admit your finger, gently insert it into the canal and ask the person to bear down. Normally, you will feel no change. Repeat the procedure on the other side.

Palpate the femoral area for a bulge. Normally you feel none.

Palpable herniating mass bumps your fingertip or pushes against the side of your finger (see Table 21–6 in Jarvis: *Physical Examination and Health Assessment,* p. 827).

INGUINAL LYMPH NODES

Palpate the horizontal chain along the groin inferior to the inguinal ligament and the vertical chain along the upper inner thigh.

On occasion, it is normal to palpate an isolated node. It then feels small (<1 cm), soft, discrete, and movable.

Enlarged, hard, matted, fixed nodes.

SELF-CARE—TESTICULAR SELF EXAMINATION (TSE)

Encourage self-care behaviors by instructing each male (from adolescence to adulthood) in examining his own testicles every month. The incidence of testicular cancer is not high, but such a tumor has no early symptoms. If detected early by palpation and treated, the prognosis is much improved. Early detection is enhanced if the person is familiar with the normal consistency of his testes. Phrase the teaching something like this:

A good time to examine the testicles is during the shower or bath when your hands and scrotum are warm. Cold hands stimulate a muscle (cremasteric) reflex, retracting the scrotal contents. The procedure is simple. Hold the scrotum in the palm of your hand and gently feel each testicle using your thumb and first two fingers. If it hurts, you are using too much pressure. The testi-

NORMAL RANGE OF FINDINGS   ABNORMAL FINDINGS

cle is egg-shaped and movable. It feels rubbery with a smooth surface. The epididymis is on top and behind the testicle; it feels a bit softer. If you notice a firm, painless lump, a hard area, or an overall enlarged testicle, call your physician for a further check.

DEVELOPMENTAL CONSIDERATIONS

The Aging Adult

In the older male, you may note thinner, graying pubic hair and a decreased size of the penis. The size of the testes may be decreased and feel less firm. The scrotal sac is pendulous with less rugae. The scrotal skin may become excoriated if the man continually sits on it.

Table 17-1 ► Sex Maturity Ratings (SMR) in Boys

DEVELOPMENTAL STAGE	PUBIC HAIR	PENIS	SCROTUM
1	No pubic hair. Fine body hair on abdomen (vellus hair), continues over pubic area	Preadolescent, size and proportion the same as during childhood	Preadolescent, size and proportion the same as during childhood
2	Few straight, slightly darker hairs at base of penis. Hair is long and downy	Little or no enlargement	Testes and scrotum begin to enlarge. Scrotal skin reddens and changes in texture
3	Sparse growth over entire pubis. Hair darker, coarser and curly	Penis begins to enlarge, especially in length	Further enlarged
4	Thick growth over pubic area but not on thighs. Hair coarse and curly as in adult	Penis grows in length and diameter, with development of glans	Testes almost fully grown, scrotum darker
5	Growth spread over medial thighs, although not yet up toward umbilicus*	Adult size and shape	Adult size and shape

(Adapted from Tanner JM: Growth at Adolescence. Oxford, England, Blackwell Scientific, 1962.)

*After puberty, pubic hair growth continues until the mid-20s, extending up the abdomen toward the umbilicus.

☑ SUMMARY CHECKLIST

1 ▶ Inspect and palpate the penis.
2 ▶ Inspect and palpate the scrotum.
3 ▶ If a mass exists, note associated signs.

4 ▶ Palpate for an inguinal hernia.
5 ▶ Palpate the inguinal lymph nodes.
6 ▶ Teach testicular self-examination.

Nursing Diagnoses Commonly Associated with the Male Genitalia and Related Disorders

Altered growth and development

Altered sexuality patterns

Impaired skin integrity

Incontinence

Rape trauma response

Rape trauma syndrome: Compound reaction

Rape trauma syndrome: Silent reaction

Sexual dysfunction

Urinary retention

18 Female Genitalia

ANATOMY

EXTERNAL GENITALIA

The external genitalia are called the *vulva* or pudendum (Fig. 18–1). The labia majora and labia minora encircle a space termed the vestibule. Within this space, the urethral meatus appears as a dimple 2.5 cm posterior to the clitoris.

The vaginal orifice is posterior to the urethral meatus. On either side and posterior to the vaginal orifice

are the two Bartholin's glands, which secrete a clear lubricating mucus during intercourse.

INTERNAL GENITALIA

The *vagina* is a flattened tubular canal extending from the orifice up and backward into the pelvis (Fig. 18–2). At the end of the canal, the

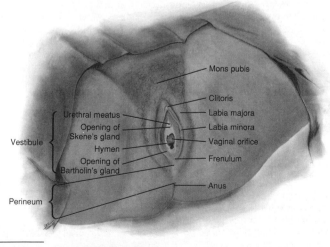

Mons pubis

Clitoris

Labia majora

Urethral meatus

Labia minora

Opening of Skene's gland

Vestibule

Vaginal orifice

Hymen

Opening of Bartholin's gland

Frenulum

Anus

Perineum

▶ Figure 18–1   The External Genitalia

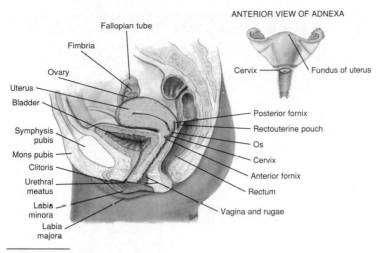

ANTERIOR VIEW OF ADNEXA

Fallopian tube

Fimbria

Ovary

Uterus

Bladder

Symphysis pubis

Mons pubis

Clitoris

Urethral meatus

Labia minora

Labia majora

Cervix — Fundus of uterus

Posterior fornix

Rectouterine pouch

Os

Cervix

Anterior fornix

Rectum

Vagina and rugae

▶ Figure 18–2   Internal genitalia

uterine *cervix* projects into the vagina.

The *uterus* is a pear-shaped, thick-walled, muscular organ. It is flattened anteroposteriorly, measuring 5.5 to 8 cm long by 3.5 to 4 cm wide and 2 to 2.5 cm thick, and is movable.

The *fallopian tubes* are two trumpet-shaped, pliable tubes, 10 cm in length, extending from the uterine fundus laterally to the brim of the pelvis with their ends near the ovaries. Each *ovary* is oval shaped, 3 cm long by 2 cm wide by 1 cm thick, and serves to develop ova (eggs) as well as the female hormones.

DEVELOPMENTAL CONSIDERATIONS

The first signs of puberty are breast and pubic hair development, beginning between the ages of 8½ and 13 years. These signs are usually concurrent, but it is not abnormal if they do not develop together. They take about 3 years to complete.

Menarche occurs during the latter half of this sequence, just after the peak of growth velocity.

Tanner's table on the five stages of pubic hair development is helpful in teaching girls the expected sequence of sexual development (see Table 18–1 on p. 227).

SUBJECTIVE DATA

Menstrual history
  Last menstrual period (LMP)
  Age at menarche
  Cycle
  Duration

Obstetric history
  Gravida—number of pregnancies
  Para—number of births.
  Abortions—interrupted pregnancies, including elective abortions and spontaneous miscarriages.

Self-care behaviors
  Gynecological checkup

Urinary symptoms
  Frequency, urgency, dysuria

Vaginal discharge—color, characteristics

Sexual activity

Contraceptive use

Sexually transmitted disease (STD) contact

O B J E C T I V E   D A T A

Equipment Needed

Assemble these items before helping the women into position. Arrange within easy reach.

Gloves—wear gloves during every female genitalia examination

Goose-necked lamp with a strong light

Vaginal speculum of appropriate size
   Graves' speculum—useful for most adult women, available in varying lengths and widths
   Pederson speculum—narrow blades, useful for virginal or postmenopausal women with a narrowed introitus

Large cotton-tipped applicators (rectal swabs)

Materials for cytologic study:
   Glass slide
   Sterile cotton-tipped applicator or endocervical brush
   Ayre's spatula
   Spray fixative

Lubricant

Preparation

Initially for the health history, the woman should be sitting up.

For the examination, the woman should be placed in the lithotomy position, with the examiner sitting on a stool. Help the woman into lithotomy position, with the body supine, feet in stirrups and knees apart, and buttocks at edge of examining table. The arms should be at the woman's sides or across the chest, not over the head, because this position only tightens the abdominal muscles. Drape the woman fully, covering the stomach, knees, and legs, exposing only the vulva to your view. Be sure to push down the drape between the woman's legs so that you can see her face.

You can help the woman relax, decrease her anxiety, and retain a sense of control by employing these measures.

• Have her empty the bladder before the examination.

- Elevate her head and shoulders to maintain eye contact.
- Pull out the stirrups so the legs are not abducted too far.
- Explain each step in the examination before you do it.
- Assure the woman she can stop the examination at any point should she feel any discomfort.
- Touch the inner thigh before you touch the vulva.
- Communicate throughout the examination. Maintain a dialogue to share information.

METHOD OF EXAMINATION

NORMAL RANGE OF FINDINGS	ABNORMAL FINDINGS

EXTERNAL GENITALIA

Inspect the External Genitalia Noting:

- Skin color.
- Hair distribution is in the usual female pattern of inverted triangle, although it may normally trail up the abdomen toward the umbilicus.

Consider delayed puberty if no pubic hair or breast development has occurred by age 13.
   Nits or lice at the base of pubic hair.

- Labia major are normally symmetric, plump, and well formed. In the nulliparous woman, labia meet in the midline; following a vaginal delivery, the labia are gaping and slightly shriveled.

Swelling.

- There should be no lesions, except for occasional sebaceous cysts. These are yellowish, 1-cm nodules that are firm, nontender, and often multiple.

Excoriation.
Nodules.
Rash or lesions (Table 22–3 in Jarvis: *Physical Examination and Health Assessment*, p. 863).

   With your gloved hand, separate the labia majora to inspect:

- Clitoris.

Enlarged clitoris.

- Labia minora are dark pink and moist, usually symmetric.

Inflammation.

- Urethral opening appears stellate or slitlike and is midline.

Polyp.

- Vaginal opening, or introitus, may appear as a narrow vertical slit or as a larger opening.

Rash or lesions.
   Foul smelling, irritating, or yellow, white or gray discharge.

NORMAL RANGE OF FINDINGS	ABNORMAL FINDINGS

- Perineum is smooth. A well-healed episiotomy scar, midline or medio-lateral, may be present following a vaginal birth.
- Anus has coarse skin of increased pigmentation (see Chapter 19 for assessment).

Palpate Glands

Assess urethra and Skene's glands. Insert your index finger into the va-gina, and gently milk the urethra by applying pressure up and out. This procedure should produce no pain. If any discharge appears, culture it.

Tenderness.
Induration along urethra.
Urethral discharge.

Assess Bartholin's glands. Palpate the posterior parts of the labia ma-jora with your index finger in the vagina and your thumb outside (Fig. 18–3). The labia normally feel soft and homogeneous.

Swelling.
Induration.
Pain with palpation.
Discharge from duct opening.

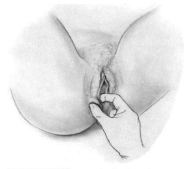

▶ Figure 18–3   Palpate labia majora

Assess the Support of Pelvic Musculature:

- Palpate the perineum. It normally feels thick, smooth, and muscular in the nulliparous woman and thin and rigid in the multiparous woman.

Tenderness.
Paper-thin perineum.

- Using your index and middle fingers, separate the vaginal orifice and ask the woman to strain down. There normally is no bulg-ing of vaginal walls or urinary in-continence.

Bulging of the vaginal wall indi-cates cystocele, rectocele, or uter-ine prolapse (see Table 22–4 in Jarvis: *Physical Examination and Health Assessment,* p. 866).
    Urinary incontinence.

NORMAL RANGE OF FINDINGS	ABNORMAL FINDINGS

INTERNAL GENITALIA

Speculum Examination

Select the proper-sized speculum. Warm and lubricate the speculum under warm, running water. Avoid gel lubricant at this point because it is bacteriostatic and would distort cells in the cytology specimen you will collect.

Hold the speculum in your right hand with the index and the middle fingers surrounding the blades and your thumb under the thumbscrew. This prevents the blades from opening painfully during insertion. With your left index and middle fingers, push the introitus down and open (Fig. 18–4). Tilt the width of the blades obliquely and insert the speculum past your left fingers, applying any pressure downward. This avoids pressure on the anterior vaginal wall and on the sensitive urethra above it.

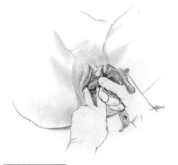

▶ Figure 18–4   Insert vaginal speculum

Ease insertion by asking the woman to bear down. This method relaxes the perineal muscles and opens the introitus.

As the blades pass your left fingers, withdraw your fingers. Now turn the width of the blades horizontally, and continue to insert in a 45-degree angle downward toward the small of the woman's back. This

NORMAL RANGE OF FINDINGS	ABNORMAL FINDINGS

matches the natural slope of the vagina.

After the blades are fully inserted, open them by squeezing the handles together (Fig. 18–5). The cervix should be in full view. Lock the blades open by tightening the thumbscrew.

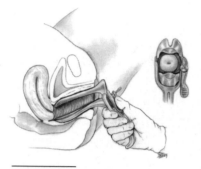

▶ Figure 18–5   Open speculum blades and view cervix

Inspect the Cervix and Its Os. Note:

1. Color. Normally, the cervical mucosa is pink and even. During the second month of pregnancy it looks blue (Chadwick's sign), and after menopause it is pale.

    Redness, inflammation.
    Pallor with anemia.
    Cyanotic other than with pregnancy (see Table 22–5 in Jarvis: *Physical Examination and Health Assessment*, p. 867).

2. Position. Midline, either anterior or posterior. Projects 1 to 3 cm into the vagina.
3. Size. Diameter is 2.5 cm (1 inch).
4. Os. This is small and round in the nulliparous woman. In the parous woman, it is a horizontal irregular slit and also may show healed lacerations on the sides.

    Surface reddened, granular and any lesion. See erosion, polyp, carcinoma, Table 22–5 in Jarvis: *Physical Examination and Health Assessment*, p. 867.

5. Surface. This is normally smooth.
6. Note cervical secretions. Depending on the day of the menstrual cycle, secretions may be clear and thin, or thick, opaque, and stringy. They are always odorless and nonirritating.

    Foul-smelling, irritating, or yellow, green, white, or gray discharge (see Table 22–6 in Jarvis: *Physical Examination and Health Assessment*, p. 868).

NORMAL RANGE OF FINDINGS	ABNORMAL FINDINGS

If secretions are copious, swab the area with a thick-tipped rectal swab. This method sponges away secretions, giving you a better view of the structures.

Obtain Cervical Smears and Cultures

The Papanicolaou, or Pap, smear screens for cervical cancer. Instruct the woman not to douche within 24 hours before collecting the specimens. The test requires three specimens:

Endocervical Swab. (Fig. 18–6). Insert a premoistened* cotton applicator or endocervical brush into the os and rotate it 360 degrees. Roll the swab gently on a glass slide to deposit all the cells. Avoid leaving a thick specimen that would be hard to read under the microscope. Immediately spray all slides with fixative to avoid drying.

Cervical Scrape. Insert the curved end of an Ayre spatula into the cervical os. Rotate it 360 degrees. The spatula scrapes the surface of the cervix as you turn the instrument. Spread the specimen from both sides of the spatula onto a glass slide. Use a single stroke to thin out the specimen, not a back-and-forth motion.

Vaginal Pool. Reverse the spatula and gently rub the blunt end over the vaginal wall under and lateral to the cervix. Wipe the specimen on a slide. If the mucosa is very dry (as in a postmenopausal woman), moisten a sterile swab with normal saline to collect this specimen.

---

*Premoistening the applicator with normal saline prevents the sample cells from being absorbed into the cotton, and it prevents the cotton threads from distorting the specimen.

NORMAL RANGE OF FINDINGS	ABNORMAL FINDINGS

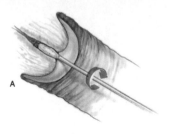

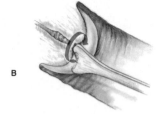

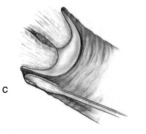

▶ Figure 18–6 Pap smear specimens:
(A) Endocervical swab,
(B) Cervical scrape,
(C) Vaginal pool.

Inspect the Vaginal Wall

Loosen the thumbscrew but continue to hold the speculum blades open. Slowing withdraw the speculum, rotating it as you go, to fully inspect the vaginal wall. Normally, the wall looks pink, deeply rugated, moist and smooth, and is free of inflammation or lesions. Normal discharge is thin and clear, or opaque and stringy, but always odorless.

Reddened.
Pallor prior to menopause.
Lesions.
Vaginal discharge: Thick, any gray, green-yellow, white or foul-smelling discharge (see Table 22–6 in Jarvis: *Physical Examination and Health Assessment*, p. 868).

NORMAL RANGE OF FINDINGS

ABNORMAL FINDINGS

When the blades end near the vaginal opening, let them close, but be careful not to pinch the mucosa or catch any hairs. Turn the blades obliquely to avoid stretching the opening. Clean the metal speculum and place it in a soaking solution; discard the plastic variety.

Bimanual Examination

Use both hands to palpate the internal genitalia to assess their location, size, and mobility, and to screen for any tenderness or mass. One hand is on the abdomen while the other (often the dominant, more sensitive hand) inserts two fingers into the vagina.

Rise to a stand, and have the woman remain in lithotomy position. Glove and lubricate the first two fingers of your intravaginal hand. Insert your fingers into the vagina, with any pressure directed posteriorly.

Palpate the Internal Genitalia

Palpate the vaginal wall. It normally feels smooth and has no area of induration or tenderness.

Locate the cervix in the midline, often near the anterior vaginal wall. Note these characteristics of a normal cervix:

- Consistency—feels smooth and firm, as the consistency of the tip of the nose. It softens and feels velvety at 5 to 6 weeks of pregnancy (Goodell's sign).

- Contour—evenly rounded.

- Mobility—With a finger on either side, move the cervix gently from side to side. Normally, this produces no pain (Fig. 18–7).

Palpate all around the fornices; the wall should feel smooth.

Next, use your abdominal hand to push the pelvic organs closer for your intravaginal fingers to palpate. Place your hand midway between the umbilicus and the symphysis;

Nodule.
Tenderness.

Hard with malignancy.
Nodular.

Irregular.

Immobile with malignancy.
Painful with inflammation or ectopic pregnancy.

Nodular.
Irregular.

NORMAL RANGE OF FINDINGS	ABNORMAL FINDINGS

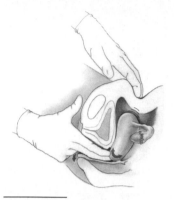

▶ Figure 18–7   Palpate the cervix

push down in a slow, firm manner, fingers together and slightly flexed.

With your intravaginal fingers in the anterior fornix, assess the uterus. Determine the position, or *version*, of the uterus. In many women, the uterus is anteverted; you palpate it at the level of the pubis with the cervix pointing posteriorly. Two other positions normally occur (midposition and retroverted), as well as two aspects of flexion, where the long axis of the uterus is not straight but flexed (for illustration, see Fig. 22-19, p. 852 in Jarvis: *Physical Examination and Health Assessment*).

Palpate the uterine wall with your fingers in the fornices. It normally feels firm and smooth, with the contour of the fundus rounded. It softens during pregnancy. Bounce the uterus gently between your abdominal and intravaginal hand. It should be freely movable and nontender.

Move both hands to the right to explore the adnexa. Place your abdominal hand on the lower quadrant just inside the anterior iliac spine with your intravaginal fingers in the lateral fornix (Fig. 18–8). Push the abdominal hand in and try to capture the ovary. You often cannot feel the ovary. When you can, it

Enlarged uterus (see Table 22–7, pp. 870–871 in Jarvis: *Physical Examination and Health Assessment*).
Lateral displacement.
Nodular mass.
Irregular, asymmetric.
Fixed.
Tenderness.

NORMAL RANGE OF FINDINGS

ABNORMAL FINDINGS

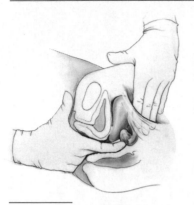

▶ Figure 18–8   Palpate the adnexa

normally feels smooth, firm, almond-shaped, and is highly movable, sliding through the fingers. It is slightly sensitive but not painful. The fallopian tube is not normally palpable. There should be no other mass or pulsation.

A note of caution—normal adnexal structures are often not palpable. To be safe, any mass that you cannot *positively* identify as a normal structure, should be considered abnormal, and the woman referred for further study.

Move to the left to palpate the other side. Then withdraw your hand and check secretions on the fingers before discarding the glove. Normal secretions are clear or cloudy and odorless.

Rectovaginal Examination

Use this technique to assess the rectovaginal septum, posterior uterine wall, cul-de-sac, and rectum. Change gloves to avoid spreading any possible infection. Lubricate the first two fingers. Tell the woman this may feel uncomfortable and will mimic the feeling of moving

Enlarged adnexa.
Nodular.
Immobile.
Markedly tender.
Mass.

Pulsation or palpable fallopian tube suggests ectopic pregnancy. Warrants immediate referral (see Table 22–8, pp. 872–873 in Jarvis: *Physical Examination and Health Assessment*).

NORMAL RANGE OF FINDINGS	ABNORMAL FINDINGS

her bowels. Ask her to bear down as you insert your index finger into the vagina and your middle finger gently into the rectum (Figure 18–9).

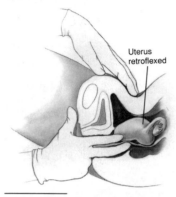

Uterus retroflexed

▶ Figure 18–9   Rectovaginal palpation

While pushing with the abdominal hand, repeat the steps of the bimanual exam. Try to keep the intravaginal finger on the cervix so the intrarectal finger does not mistake the cervix for a mass. Note:

• Rectovaginal septum should feel smooth, thin, firm, and pliable.

Nodular.
Thickened.

• Rectovaginal pouch, or cul-de-sac, is a potential space and usually not palpated.

• Uterine wall and fundus feel firm and smooth.

Rotate the intrarectal finger to check the rectal wall and anal sphincter tone. (See Chapter 19 for Assessment of Anus and Rectum). Check your gloved finger as you withdraw; test any adherent stool for occult blood.

Give the woman tissues to wipe the area and help her up. Remind her to slide her hips back from the table edge before sitting up so she will not fall.

NORMAL RANGE OF FINDINGS	ABNORMAL FINDINGS

DEVELOPMENTAL CONSIDERATIONS

The Pregnant Female

The external genitalia show hyperemia of the perineum and vulva because of increased vascularity. Varicose veins may be visible in the labia or legs. Hemorrhoids may show around the anus. Both are caused by interruption in venous return from the pressure of the fetus.

Internally, the walls of the vagina appear violet or blue owing to hyperemia. The vaginal walls are deeply rugated and vaginal mucosa thickens. The cervix looks blue and feels velvety and softer than in the nonpregnant state, making it a bit more difficult to differentiate from the vaginal walls.

During bimanual examination, the isthmus of the uterus feels softer and is more easily compressed between your two hands (Hegar's sign). The fundus balloons between your two hands; it feels connected to, but distinct from, the cervix because the isthmus is so soft.

Search the adnexal area carefully during early pregnancy. Normally, the adnexal structures are not palpable.

An ectopic pregnancy has serious consequences (see Table 22–8 in Jarvis: *Physical Examination and Health Assessment*, p. 872).

The Aging Adult

Natural lubrication is decreased; to avoid a painful examination, take care to lubricate instruments and the examining hand adequately.

Menopause and the resulting decrease in estrogen production shows numerous physical changes. Pubic hair gradually decreases, becoming thin and sparse in later years. Fat deposits decrease, leaving the mons pubis smaller and the labia flatter. Clitoris size also decreases after age 60.

Internally, the rugae of the vaginal walls decrease, and the walls look pale pink because of the

NORMAL RANGE OF FINDINGS	ABNORMAL FINDINGS

thinned epithelium. The cervix shrinks and looks pale and glistening. It may retract, appearing to be flush with the vaginal wall. In some, it is hard to distinguish the cervix from the surrounding vaginal mucosa. Alternately, the cervix may protrude into the vagina if the uterus has prolapsed.

With the bimanual examination, the uterus feels smaller and firmer, and the ovaries are not normally palpable.

Table 18–1 ► Sex Maturity Rating (SMR) in Girls

STAGE	DESCRIPTION	
1	Preadolescent. No pubic hair. Mons and labia covered with fine vellus hair as on abdomen.	
2	Growth sparse and mostly on labia. Long downy hair, slightly pigmented, straight or only slightly curly.	
3	Growth sparse and spreading over mons pubis. Hair is darker, coarser, curlier.	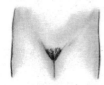
4	Hair is adult in type but over smaller area; none on medial thigh	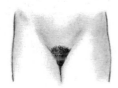
5	Adult in type and pattern; inverse triangle. Also on medial thigh surface.	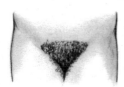

(Adapted from Tanner JM: Growth at Adolescence. Oxford, England, Blackwell Scientific, 1962.)

☑ SUMMARY CHECKLIST

1 ▶ Inspect external genitalia.
2 ▶ Palpate labia, Skene's and Bartholin's glands.
3 ▶ Using vaginal speculum, inspect cervix and vagina.
4 ▶ Obtain specimens for cytologic study.

5 ▶ Perform bimanual examination: cervix, uterus, adnexa.
6 ▶ Perform rectovaginal examination.
7 ▶ Test stool for occult blood.

Nursing Diagnoses Commonly Associated with the Female Genitalia and Related Disorders

Altered growth and development

Altered sexuality patterns

Functional incontinence

Impaired skin integrity

Pain

Rape-trauma response

Reflex incontinence

Sexual dysfunction

Stress incontinence

Total incontinence

Urge incontinence

CHAPTER

19 Anus, Rectum and Prostate

ANATOMY

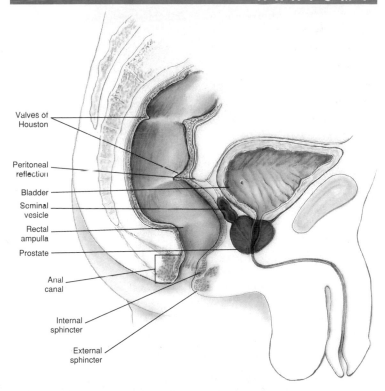

Valves of
Houston

Peritoneal
reflection

Bladder

Seminal
vesicle

Rectal
ampulla

Prostate

Anal
canal

Internal
sphincter

External
sphincter

▶ Figure 19-1   The anal canal, rectum, and male prostate

The *anal canal* is the outlet of the gastrointestinal tract and is about 3.8 cm long in the adult (Fig. 19–1). It slants forward toward the umbilicus, forming a distinct right angle with the rectum, which rests back in the hollow of the sacrum.

The anal canal is surrounded by two concentric layers of muscle, the *internal* and *external sphincters.*

The *rectum,* which is 12 cm long, is the distal portion of the large intestine. Just above the anal canal,

the rectum dilates, and turns posteriorly, forming the rectal ampulla.

In the male, the *prostate gland* lies in front of the anterior wall of the rectum. It surrounds the bladder neck and the urethra, and it secretes a thin milky alkaline fluid that helps sperm viability. It has two lobes that are separated by a shallow groove called the *median sulcus.* The two *seminal vesicles* project like rabbit ears above the prostate.

SUBJECTIVE DATA

Usual bowel routine: frequency, stool color

Change in bowel habits: diarrhea, constipation, use of enemas

Medications: laxatives, stool softeners, iron

Rectal conditions (pruritus, hemorrhoids, fissure, fistula)

Diet of high-fiber foods

OBJECTIVE DATA

Equipment Needed

Penlight

Lubricating jelly

Glove

Guaiac test reagents

Preparation

Examine the male in the left lateral decubitus position or standing and leaning over an exam table. Place the female in lithotomy position if examining genitalia as well; use the left lateral decubitus position for the rectal area alone.

METHOD OF EXAMINATION

NORMAL RANGE OF FINDINGS	ABNORMAL FINDINGS

EXAMINATION OF THE ANAL REGION

Inspect the Perianal Area

The anus normally appears moist and hairless, with coarse, folded, pigmented skin. The anal opening is tightly closed. There are no lesions.

Inflammation.
Lesions or scars.
Linear split — fissure.
Flabby skin sac — hemorrhoid.
　Shiny blue skin sac — thrombosed hemorrhoid.
　Small round opening in anal area — fistula.

The sacrococcygeal area appears smooth and even.

Inflammation or tenderness, swelling, tuft of hair, or dimple at tip of coccyx may indicate pilonidal cyst (see Table 23–1 in Jarvis: *Physical Examination and Health Assessment*, pp. 891–892).
Appearance of fissure.
Appearance of hemorrhoids.
　Circular red doughnut of tissue — rectal prolapse.

Instruct the person to hold his or her breath and bear down by performing a Valsalva maneuver. There should be no break in skin integrity or protrusion through the anal opening.

Palpate the Anus and Rectum

Don a glove and drop lubricating jelly onto your index finger. Inform the person that palpation is not painful but may feel as if needing to move the bowels.

Place the pad of your index finger gently against the anal verge. You will feel the sphincter tighten, then relax. As it relaxes, flex the tip of your finger and slowly insert it into the anal canal in a direction toward the umbilicus.

Rotate your examining finger to palpate the entire muscular ring. The canal should feel smooth and even. To assess tone, ask the person to tighten the muscle. The sphincter should tighten evenly around your finger with no pain to the person.

Above the anal canal, the rectum turns posteriorly, following the

Decreased tone.
　Increased tone occurs with inflammation and anxiety.
Thrombosed internal hemorrhoid.

NORMAL RANGE OF FINDINGS	ABNORMAL FINDINGS

curve of the coccyx and sacrum. Insert your finger farther and explore all around the rectal wall. It normally feels smooth with no nodularity. Promptly report any mass you discover for further examination.

A soft, slightly moveable mass may be a polyp.

A firm or hard mass with irregular shape or rolled edges may signify carcinoma (see Table 23–2 in Jarvis: *Physical Examination and Health Assessment*, p. 893).

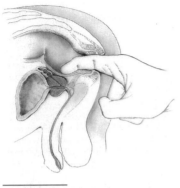

► Figure 19–2   Palpate the prostate gland

Palpate the Prostate Gland

In the male, palpate the prostate gland on the anterior wall (Fig. 19–2). Note:

Size	2.5 cm long by 4 cm wide. Should not protrude more than 1 cm into the rectum.
Shape	Heart shaped, with palpable central groove.
Surface	Smooth.
Consistency	Elastic, rubbery.
Mobility	Slightly moveable.
Sensitivity	Nontender to palpation.

Enlarged or atrophied gland.

Flat with no groove.

Nodular
Hard, boggy, soft, fluctuant.
Fixed.
Tender.

Enlarged, firm, smooth gland with central groove obliterated suggests benign prostatic hypertrophy (BPH).

Swollen, exquisitely tender gland accompanies prostatitis.

Any stone-hard, irregular, fixed nodule indicates carcinoma (see Table 23–3 in Jarvis: *Physical Examination and Health Assessment*, p. 894).

NORMAL RANGE OF FINDINGS

Withdraw your examining finger; normally, there is no bright red blood or mucus on the glove. Offer the person tissues to remove the lubricant and help the person to a more comfortable position.

Examination of Stool. Inspect any feces remaining on the glove. Normally, the color is brown and consistency is soft.

Test any stool on the glove for *occult* (or hidden) *blood.* Use the *guaiac test* to detect small quantities of blood. A negative response is normal. If the stool is *guaiac positive,* it indicates occult blood. Note that a false-positive finding may occur if the person has ingested significant amounts of red meat within 3 days of the test.

ABNORMAL FINDINGS

Jelly-like mucus shreds mixed in stool indicate inflammation.

Bright red blood on stool surface indicates rectal bleeding. Bright red blood mixed with feces indicates possible colonic bleeding.

Black tarry stool with distinct malodor indicates upper gastrointestinal bleeding, with blood partially digested.

Black stool—also occurs with ingesting iron medications or bismuth preparations.

Gray, tan stool—occurs with absent bile pigment, e.g., obstructive jaundice.

Pale yellow, greasy, stool—increased fat content (steatorrhea), as occurs with malabsorption syndrome.

Occult bleeding usually indicates cancer of colon.

☑ SUMMARY CHECKLIST

1 ▶ Inspect anus and perianal area.
2 ▶ Inspect during Valsalva maneuver.

3 ▶ Palpate anal canal and rectum on all adults.
4 ▶ Test stool for occult blood.

Nursing Diagnoses Commonly Associated with Anal and Rectal Disorders

Bowel incontinence

Colonic constipation

Constipation

Diarrhea

Perceived constipation

Skin integrity, impaired

20 Integration of the Complete Physical Examination

The following examination sequence combines all the separate steps into a complete and smoothly flowing assessment. The sequence clusters steps by body region and proceeds systematically head-to-toe, concluding with examination of the genitalia. This is the most efficient way of conducting the examination, and it minimizes the number of position changes for you and the client, thus avoiding tiring the client. The running second column presents a sample recording when findings are within the normal range.

Sequence	Sample Recording

The person walks into the room, sits; the examiner sits facing the client; the client is in street clothes.

THE HEALTH HISTORY

1. Collect the history, complete or limited as visit warrants. While obtaining the history and throughout the examination, note data on the person's general appearance.

GENERAL APPEARANCE

1. Appears stated age.
2. Level of consciousness.
3. Skin color.
4. Nutritional status.
5. Posture and position comfortably erect.
6. Obvious physical deformities.

(Client's name) is a (age)-year-old (male/female), well nourished, well developed, who appears stated age. (S)he is alert, oriented, cooperative, with no signs of acute distress. Appearance, behavior, and speech are appropriate; recent and remote memory intact.

Sequence	Sample Recording

7. Mobility.
    Gait
    Use of assistive devices
    Range of motion of joints
    No involuntary movement
8. Facial expression.
9. Mood and affect.
10. Speech: articulation, pattern, content appropriate, native language
11. Hearing.
12. Personal hygiene.

MEASUREMENT

1. Weight.
2. Height.
3. Skinfold thickness, if indicated.
4. Vision using Snellen eye chart.

Weight   57 kg   (126 lbs),   height 163 cm   (5′4″),   skinfold thickness 20 mm,   vision O.D. 20/20, O.S. 20/30 −1.

Ask the client to empty the bladder (save specimen, if needed), disrobe except for underpants, and put on a gown. The client sits with legs dangling off side of the bed or table; examiner stands in front of the person.

SKIN

1. Examine both hands and inspect the nails.
2. For the rest of the examination, examine skin with corresponding regional examination.

Skin. Color tan-pink (light brown, brown, brown-black), warm to touch; turgor good, no lesions. Nails: No clubbing or deformities, nailbeds pink with prompt capillary refill.

VITAL SIGNS

1. Radial pulse.
2. Respirations.
3. Blood pressure.
4. Temperature.

TPR: 37°C–76–14,   BP   128/84 right arm, sitting.

HEAD AND FACE

1. Inspect and palpate scalp, hair, and cranium.
2. Inspect fact: expression, symmetry (cranial nerve VII).
3. Palpate the temporal artery, then the temporomandibular joint as the client opens and closes the mouth.

Hair: texture fine, distribution appropriate for age.
Head: Normocephalic, no lumps, no lesions, no tenderness.
Face: Symmetric, no weakness, n involuntary movements.

Sequence	Sample Recording

4. Palpate the maxillary sinuses and the frontal sinuses; if tender, transilluminate the sinuses.

EYES

1. Test visual fields by confrontation (cranial nerve II).
2. Test extraocular muscles: corneal light reflex, 6 cardinal positions of gaze (cranial nerves III, IV, VI).
3. Inspect external eye structures.
4. Inspect conjunctivae, sclerae, corneae, irides.
5. Test pupils: size, response to light and accommodation.

Darken room.

6. Using an ophthalomoscope, inspect ocular fundus: red reflex, disc, vessels, and retinal background.

Eyes: Visual fields intact by confrontation. EOMs intact. Brows and lashes present. No ptosis. Conjunctivae clear. Sclerae white, no lesions. PERRLA.
Fundi: Red reflex present bilaterally. Discs flat with sharp margins. Vessels persent in all quadrants without crossing defects. Retinal background has even color with no hemorrhages or exudates. Macula has even color.

EARS

1. Inspect the external ear: position and alignment, skin condition, and auditory meatus.
2. Move auricle and push tragus for tenderness.
3. Using an otoscope, inspect the canal then the tympanic membrane for color, position, landmarks, and integrity.
4. Test hearing: voice test, tuning fork tests—Weber and Rinne.

Ears: No masses, lesions, tenderness, or discharge. Both TMs pearly gray with light reflex and landmarks intact, no perforations. Whispered words heard bilaterally. Weber midline with lateralization. Rinne AC > BC and = bilaterally.

NOSE

1. Inspect the external nose: symmetry, lesions.
2. Test the patency of each nostril.
3. Using a nasal speculum, inspect the nares: nasal mucosa, septum, and turbinates.

Nose: No deformity. Nares patent. Mucosa pink, no septal deviation or perforation.

MOUTH AND THROAT

1. Using a penlight inspect the mouth: buccal mucosa, teeth and gums, tongue, floor of mouth, palate, and uvula.
2. Grade tonsils, if present.

Mouth: Can clench teeth. Mucosa and gingivae pink, no masses or lesions. Teeth in good repair. Tongue protrudes in midline, no tremor.

Sequence	Sample Recording
3. Note mobility of uvula as the client phonates "ahh" and test gag reflex (cranial nerves IX, X).	*Throat: Mucosa pink, no lesions. Uvula arises in midline on phonation. Tonsils out. Gag reflex present.*
4. Ask the person to stick out the tongue (cranial nerve XII).	
5. Palpate the mouth bimanually if indicated.	

NECK

1. Inspect the neck: symmetry, lumps, and pulsations.	*Neck: Supple with full ROM, no pain. Symmetric, no lymphadenopathy or masses; trachea midline; thyroid not palpable, no bruits. Carotid pulses 2+ and = bilaterally.*
2. Palpate the cervical lymph nodes.	
3. Inspect and palpate the carotid pulse, one side at a time. If indicated, listen for carotid bruits.	
4. Palpate the trachea in midline.	
5. Test range of motion and muscle strength against your resistance: head forward and back, head turned to each side, and shoulder shrug (cranial nerve XI).	

Step behind the person, taking your stethoscope, ruler, and marking pen with you.

6. Palpate thyroid gland.

Open the person's gown to expose all of the back, but leave gown on shoulders and anterior chest.

CHEST, POSTERIOR AND LATERAL

1. Inspect the posterior chest: configuration of the thoracic cage, skin characteristics, and symmetry of shoulders and muscles.	*Chest: AP < transverse diameter. Respirations 16 per minute, relaxed and even. Chest expansion symmetric. Tactile fremitus equal bilaterally. Resonant to percussion over lung fields. Diaphragmatic excursion 5 cm and = bilaterally. Breath sounds clear. No adventitious sounds.*
2. Palpate: symmetric expansion, tactile fremitus, lumps, or tenderness.	
3. Palpate length of spinous processes.	
4. Percuss over all lung fields, noting diaphragmatic excursion.	
5. Percuss costovertebral angle noting tenderness.	
6. Auscultate breath sounds, note adventitious sounds.	

Sequence	Sample Recording

Move around to face the client; the client remains sitting. At the time for the female breast examination, ask client's permission to lift gown to drape on the shoulders, exposing the anterior chest; for a male, lower the gown to the lap.

ANTERIOR CHEST

1. Inspect: respirations and skin characteristics.
2. Palpate: tactile fremitus, lumps, or tenderness.
3. Percuss lung fields.
4. Auscultate breath sounds.

HEART

1. Ask the person to lean forward slightly and exhale briefly; auscultate base for any murmurs.

(See Sample Recording in HEART section following.)

UPPER EXTREMITIES

1. Test range of motion and muscle strength of hands, arms, and shoulders.
2. Palpate the epitrochlear nodes.

(See Sample Recording in LOWER EXTREMITIES section following.)

FEMALE BREASTS

1. Inspect for symmetry, mobility, and dimpling as the woman lifts arms over the head, pushes the hands on the hips, and leans forward.
2. Inspect supraclavicular and infraclavicular areas.

Breasts symmetric. No retraction, no nipple discharge, no lesions. Contour and consistency firm and homogeneous. No masses or tenderness. No lymphadenopathy.

Help the person to lie supine with head at a 30- to 45-degree angle. Stand at the person's *right* side. Drape the gown up across shoulders and place an extra sheet across lower abdomen.

3. Palpate each breast, lifting the same side arm up over head. Include the tail of Spence and areola.
4. Palpate each nipple for discharge.
5. Support the person's arm and palpate axilla and regional lymph nodes.
6. Teach breast self-examination.

Sequence	Sample Recording

MALE BREASTS

1. Inspect and palpate while palpating the anterior chest wall.
2. Supporting each arm, palpate the axilla and regional nodes.

NECK VESSELS

1. Inspect each side of neck for a jugular venous pulse, turning the person's head slightly to the other side.
2. Estimate the jugular venous pressure, if indicated.

External jugular veins flat.

HEART

1. Inspect the precordium for pulsations and heave (lift).
2. Palpate the apical impulse, and note the location.
3. Palpate precordium for thrills.
4. Auscultate apical rate and rhythm.
5. Auscultate with the diaphragm of the stethoscope to study heart sounds, inching from the apex up to the base, or vice versa.
6. Auscultate the heart sounds with the bell of the stethoscope, again inching through all locations.
7. Turn the person over to left side while again auscultating apex with the bell.

Precordium: Apical impulse at 5th intercostal space, left midclavicular line. No heave or thrill, rate 68 per minute and regular, S_1 and S_2 normal, no extra sounds, no murmurs.

The person should be supine, with the bed or table flat; arrange drapes to expose the abdomen from the chest to the pubis.

ABDOMEN

1. Inspect: contour, symmetry, skin characteristics, umbilicus, and pulsations.
2. Auscultate bowel sounds.
3. Auscultate for vascular sounds over the aorta and renal arteries.
4. Percuss all quadrants.
5. Percuss height of the liver span in right midclavicular line.
6. Percuss the location of the spleen.

Abdomen: Flat, symmetric with no apparent masses. Skin smooth with no striae, scars, or lesions. Bowel sounds present, no bruits. Tympany to percussion in all 4 quadrants. Liver span 8 cm in right midclavicular line; splenic dullness at 10th intercostal space in left midaxillary line. Abdomen soft to palpation, no organomegaly, no masses, no tenderness.

Sequence	Sample Recording

7. Palpate: light palpation in all quadrants, then deep palpation in all quadrants.
8. Palpate for liver, for spleen, for kidneys, and for aorta pulsation.
9. Test the abdominal reflexes, if indicated.

INGUINAL AREA

1. Palpate each groin for the femoral pulse and the inguinal nodes.

Lift the drape to expose the legs.

LOWER EXTREMITIES

1. Inspect: symmetry, skin characteristics, and hair distribution.
2. Palpate pulses: popliteal, posterior tibial, dorsalis pedis.
3. Palpate for temperature and pretibial edema.
4. Separate toes and inspect.
5. Test range of motion and muscle strength of hips, knees, ankles, and feet.

Extremities have pink-tan (brown, brown-black) color with no redness, cyanosis, or any skin lesions. Extremity size symmetric with no swelling or atrophy. Temperature warm and = bilaterally. All pulses present, 2+ and = bilaterally. No lymphadenopathy.
(See MUSCULOSKELETAL section below for muscle sample recording.)

Ask the client to sit up and dangle the legs off the bed or table. Keep the gown on, and drape it over the lap.

MUSCULOSKELETAL

1. Note muscle strength as person performs the sit-up.

NEUROLOGIC

(Note: Cranial nerve II-XII testing was integrated during head and neck regional examinations.)
1. Test sensation in selected areas on face, arms, hands, legs, and feet: superficial pain, light touch, and vibration.
2. Test position sense of finger, one hand.
3. Test stereognosis.
4. Test cerebellar function of the upper extremities using finger-to-nose test or rapid alternating movements test.

Neurologic, sensory: Pinprick, light touch, vibration intact. Stereognosis — able to identify key.
Motor: No atrophy, weakness or tremors. RAM (rapid alternating movements) — finger-to-nose smoothly intact.
Reflexes: Normal abdominal, DTRs all 2+ and equal bilaterally, no Babinski's sign.

Sequence	Sample Recording

5. Test the cerebellar function of the lower extremities by asking the person to run each heel down the opposite shin.
6. Elicit deep tendon reflexes: biceps, triceps, brachioradialis, patellar, and Achilles.
7. Test the Babinski reflex.

Ask the client to stand with the gown on. Stand close to the client.

LOWER EXTREMITIES

1. Inspect lower legs for varicose veins.

MUSCULOSKELETAL

1. Ask the person to walk across the room, turn, then walk back toward you in heel-to-toe fashion.
2. Ask the person to walk on the toes for a few steps, then to walk on the heels for a few steps.
3. Stand close, and check the Romberg sign.
4. Ask the person to hold the edge of the bed and to perform a shallow knee bend, one for each leg.
5. Stand behind and check the spine as the person touches the toes.
6. Stabilize the pelvis and test range of motion of the spine as the person hyperextends, rotates, and laterally bends.

Musculoskeletal: Gait normal, able to tandem walk, no Romberg's sign. Joints and muscles symmetric; no swelling masses, or deformity; normal spinal curvature. No tenderness to palpation of joints; no heat, swelling, or masses. Full ROM; movement smooth, no crepitance, no tenderness. Muscle strength— able to maintain flexion against resistance and without tenderness.

Sit on a stool in front of a male. The male stands.

MALE GENITALIA

1. Inspect the penis and scrotum.
2. Palpate the scrotal contents. If a mass exists, transilluminate.
3. Check for inguinal hernia.
4. Teach testicular self-examination.

Male genitalia: No lesions, inflammation or discharge from penis. Scrotum—testes descended, symmetric, no masses. No inguinal hernia.

For an adult male, ask him to bend over the examination table, supporting the torso with forearms on the table. Assist the bedfast male to a left lateral position with the right leg drawn up. The examiner stands.

Sequence	Sample Recording

MALE RECTUM

1. Inspect the perianal area.
2. With a gloved, lubricated finger, palpate the rectal walls and prostate gland.
3. Save a stool specimen for guaiac test.

Rectum: No fissure, hemorrhoids, fistula, or skin lesions in perianal area. Sphincter tone good, no prolapse. Rectal walls smooth, no masses or tenderness. Prostate not enlarged, no masses or tenderness. Stool brown, guaiac negative.

Assist the female back to the examination table and help her assume the lithotomy position. Drape her appropriately. Examiner sits on a stool at the foot of the table, then stands.

FEMALE GENITALIA

1. Inspect the perineal and perianal areas.
2. Using a vaginal speculum, inspect the cervix and vaginal walls.
3. Procure specimens.
4. Perform a bimanual examination: cervix, uterus, and adnexa.
5. Continue the bimanual examination, checking the rectum and rectovaginal walls.
6. Save a stool specimen for guaiac test.
7. Wipe the perineal area with tissues and help the female up to a sitting position.

External genitalia: No swelling, lesions or discharge. No urethral swelling or discharge. Internal genitalia: Vaginal walls have no bulging or lesions; cervix pink with no lesions, scant clear mucoid discharge. Bimanual: No pain on moving cervix; uterus anteflexed and anterverted. Adnexa: Ovaries not enlarged.
Rectal: No hemorrhoids, fissure or lesions, no masses or tenderness. Stool brown with guaiac test negative.

Tell the person you are finished with the examination and that you will leave the room as he or she gets dressed. Return to discuss the examination, further plans, and answer any questions. Thank the person for his or her time.

For the hospitalized person, return the bed and any room equipment to the way you found it. Make sure the call light and telephone are within easy reach.

RECORDING THE DATA

Record the data from the history and physical examination as soon after the event as possible. Memory fades as the day develops, especially

Sequence	Sample Recording

when you are responsible for the care of more than one person.

It is difficult to strike a balance between recording too little data and recording too much. It is important to remember that, from a legal perspective, if it is not documented, it was not done. Data important for the diagnosis and treatment of the person's health should be recorded as well as data that contribute to your decision-making process. This includes charting relevant normal or negative findings.

On the other hand, a listing of every assessment parameter yields an unwieldy, unworkable record. One way to keep your record complete yet succinct is to study your writing style. Use short clear phrases. Avoid redundant introductory phrases such as, "The client states that. . . . " Avoid redundant descriptions such as "no inguinal, femoral, or umbilical hernias." Just write, "no hernias."

Use simple line drawings to describe your findings. You do not need artistic talent; draw a simple sketch of a tympanic membrane, breast, abdomen, or cervix and mark your findings on it. A clear picture is worth many sentences of words.

ILLUSTRATION CREDITS

CHAPTER 4

Figure 4–2: From Brest AM, Moyer JH: Hypertension: Recent Advances. Philadelphia, Lea & Febiger, 1961. Reprinted with permission.

CHAPTER 10

Art for Table 10–1: From Tanner JM: Growth at Adolescence. Oxford, England, Blackwell Scientific, 1962.

CHAPTER 15

Figure 15–8: Copyright owned by DeWayne Dalrymple.

CHAPTER 16

Figure 16–19: From Hickey JV: Neurological and Neurosurgical Nursing. 2nd ed. Philadelphia, JB Lippincott, 1986, p 121.

CHAPTER 17

Art for Table 17–1: Adapted from Tanner JM: Growth at Adolescence. 2nd ed. Oxford, England, Blackwell Scientific, 1962.

CHAPTER 18

Art for Table 18–1: Adapted from Tanner JM: Growth at Adolescence. 2nd ed. Oxford, England, Blackwell Scientific, 1962.

REFERENCES

American Cancer Society: Cancer Facts and Figures—1991. Atlanta, GA, The American Cancer Society, 1991.

Barness LA: Manual of pediatric physical diagnosis. Chicago, Year Book Medical Publishers, 1981.

Bluestone CD, Klein JO: Otitis Media in Infants and Children. Philadelphia, WB Saunders, 1988.

Cutforth R, MacDonald CB: Heart sounds and murmurs in pregnancy. Am Heart J 71:741, 1966.

Farally MR, Moore WJ: Anatomical differences in the femur and tibia between Negroes and Caucasians and their effect on locomotion. Am J Phys Anthropol 43(1):63–69, 1975.

Garn SM: Compact bone in Chinese and Japanese. Science 143(3613):1439–1441, 1964.

Harlan WR, Harlan EA, Grillo GP: Secondary sex characteristics of girls 12 to 17 years of age: The U.S. Health Examination Survey. J Pediatr 96(6):1074–1078, 1980.

Office of Minority Health: Heart Disease, Stroke, and Minorities. Closing the Gap. Public Health Service, Department of Health and Human Services. Washington, DC, Government Printing Office, 1990, pp 1–5.

Overfield T: Biologic Variation in Health and Illness: Race Age, and Sex Differences. Menlo Park, CA, Addison-Wesley Publishing, 1985.

Secretary's Task Force on Black & Minority Health: Report. Volume III: Cancer. Washington DC, U.S. Department of Health and Human Services, 1986.

Tanner JM: Growth at Adolescence. 2nd ed. Oxford, England, Blackwell Scientific, 1962.

INDEX

Note: Page numbers in *italics* refer to illustrations; page numbers followed by t refer to tables.